To: Felicity

From: Ralph Ankerman, M.D.

Mental Retardation:
Developing Pharmacotherapies

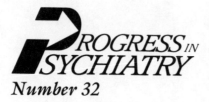

Number 32

David Spiegel, M.D.
Series Editor

Mental Retardation: Developing Pharmacotherapies

Edited by
John J. Ratey, M.D.

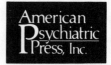

Washington, DC
London, England

Copyright © 1991 American Psychiatric Press, Inc.
ALL RIGHTS RESERVED
Manufactured in the United States of America on acid-free paper.

First Edition
94 93 92 91 4 3 2 1

American Psychiatric Press, Inc.
1400 K Street, N.W., Washington, DC 20005

Library of Congress Cataloging-in-Publication Data

Mental retardation: developing pharmacotherapies/edited by John J. Ratey.—1st ed.
    p. cm.—(Progress in psychiatry: no. 32)
  Includes bibliographical references.
  ISBN 0-88048-452-7 (alk. paper)
  1. Developmental disabilities—Chemotherapy. 2. Psychopharmacology. I. Ratey, John J., 1948-   . II. Series.
  [DNLM: 1. Mental Retardation—drug therapy. 2. Psychotropic Drugs—pharmacology. WM 300 M5493]
  RJ135.M46 1991
  616.85′88061—dc20
  DNLM/DLC
  for Library of Congress   90-14485
                                                              CIP

British Library Cataloguing in Publication Data

A CIP record is available from the British Library.

Contents

Contributors

L. Jarrett Barnhill, M.D.
Clinical Assistant Professor, University of North Carolina, Chapel Hill, North Carolina

Mark Chandler, M.D.
Assistant Professor, Department of Psychiatry/Biological Sciences Research Center, University of North Carolina, Chapel Hill, North Carolina

C. Thomas Gualtieri, M.D.
Associate Professor, Department of Psychiatry, University of North Carolina, Chapel Hill, North Carolina

Barbara H. Herman, Ph.D.
Chief, Brain Research Center, Children's National Medical Center; Associate Research Professor of Psychiatry and Behavorial Sciences and of Pediatrics, George Washington University School of Medicine, Washington, DC

Jasbir S. Kang, M.D.
Assistant Professor, University of Nebraska College of Medicine, Omaha, Nebraska

Karen J. Lindem
Research Associate, Department of Psychiatry, Harvard Medical School, Boston, Massachusetts

Frank J. Menolascino, M.D.
Chairman, Combined Department of Psychiatry, Creighton University School of Medicine and University of Nebraska College of Medicine, Omaha, Nebraska

John J. Ratey, M.D.
Assistant Professor, Department of Psychiatry, Harvard Medical School, Boston; Executive Medical Director and Director of Research, Medfield State Hospital, Medfield, Massachusetts

Edward Ritvo, M.D.
Professor, Department of Child Psychiatry, University of California, Los Angeles, School of Medicine, Los Angeles, California

Stephen L. Ruedrich, M.D.
Assistant Professor of Psychiatry, Case Western Reserve University, Cleveland, Ohio

Robert Sovner, M.D.
Developmental Disabilities/Neuropsychiatric Service, Harvard Community Health Plan, Medford, Massachusetts

Introduction to the Progress in Psychiatry Series

The Progress in Psychiatry Series is designed to capture in print the excitement that comes from assembling a diverse group of experts from various locations to examine in detail the newest information about a developing aspect of psychiatry. This series emerged as a collaboration between the American Psychiatric Association's (APA) Scientific Program Committee and the American Psychiatric Press, Inc. Great interest is generated by a number of the symposia presented each year at the APA annual meeting, and we realized that much of the information presented there, carefully assembled by people who are deeply immersed in a given area, would unfortunately not appear together in print. The symposia sessions at the annual meetings provide an unusual opportunity for experts who otherwise might not meet on the same platform to share their diverse viewpoints for a period of 3 hours. Some new themes are repeatedly reinforced and gain credence, while in other instances disagreements emerge, enabling the audience and now the reader to reach informed decisions about new directions in the field. The Progress in Psychiatry Series allows us to publish and capture some of the best of the symposia and thus provide an in-depth treatment of specific areas that might not otherwise be presented in broader review formats.

Psychiatry is by nature an interface discipline, combining the study of mind and brain, of individual and social environments, of the humane and the scientific. Therefore, progress in the field is rarely linear—it often comes from unexpected sources. Further, new developments emerge from an array of viewpoints that do not necessarily provide immediate agreement but rather expert examination of the issues. We intend to present innovative ideas and data that will enable you, the reader, to participate in this process.

We believe the Progress in Psychiatry Series will provide you with an opportunity to review timely new information in specific fields of interest as they are developing. We hope you find that the excitement of the presentations is captured in the written word and that this book proves to be informative and enjoyable reading.

David Spiegel, M.D.
Series Editor
Progress in Psychiatry Series

Progress in Psychiatry Series Titles

The Borderline: Current Empirical Research (#1)
Edited by Thomas H. McGlashan, M.D.

Premenstrual Syndrome: Current Findings and Future
Directions (#2)
Edited by Howard J. Osofsky, M.D., Ph.D., and Susan J.
Blumenthal, M.D.

Treatment of Affective Disorders in the Elderly (#3)
Edited by Charles A. Shamoian, M.D.

Post-Traumatic Stress Disorder in Children (#4)
Edited by Spencer Eth, M.D., and Robert S. Pynoos, M.D., M.P.H.

The Psychiatric Implications of Menstruation (#5)
Edited by Judith H. Gold, M.D., F.R.C.P.(C)

Can Schizophrenia Be Localized in the Brain? (#6)
Edited by Nancy C. Andreasen, M.D., Ph.D.

Medical Mimics of Psychiatric Disorders (#7)
Edited by Irl Extein, M.D., and Mark S. Gold, M.D.

Biopsychosocial Aspects of Bereavement (#8)
Edited by Sidney Zisook, M.D.

Psychiatric Pharmacosciences of Children and Adolescents (#9)
Edited by Charles Popper, M.D.

Psychobiology of Bulimia (#10)
Edited by James I. Hudson, M.D., and Harrison G. Pope, Jr., M.D.

Cerebral Hemisphere Function in Depression (#11)
Edited by Marcel Kinsbourne, M.D.

Eating Behavior in Eating Disorders (#12)
Edited by B. Timothy Walsh, M.D.

Tardive Dyskinesia: Biological Mechanisms and Clinical
Aspects (#13)
Edited by Marion E. Wolf, M.D., and Aron D. Mosnaim, Ph.D.

Current Approaches to the Prediction of Violence (#14)
Edited by David A. Brizer, M.D., and Martha L. Crowner, M.D.

Treatment of Tricyclic-Resistant Depression (#15)
Edited by Irl L. Extein, M.D.

Depressive Disorders and Immunity (#16)
Edited by Andrew H. Miller, M.D.

Chapter 1

Neuropsychiatry and Mental Retardation

John J. Ratey, M.D., and C. Thomas Gualtieri, M.D.

P sychiatry is reawakening to the need to concern itself with the subtler effects of the medications it employs. With the advent of drugs with less deleterious side effects, future research on pharmacological agents must take into account the total drug effect on patients. The field of mental retardation has been sensitized to this need for quite a few years and has helped lead the way in the search for the most effective and least cognitively impairing regimens.

Why is a new age in neuropsychiatry in order? A primary reason is that psychiatric involvement with developmentally disabled persons has radically diminished. Indeed, the psychiatric community has become largely disaffected from the developmentally disabled. Instead, the neurological community, primary-care physicians, and internists have taken over the medical care of retarded individuals. Learning theorists and educators have assumed the responsibility of constructing programs and planning treatments for this group of patients.

Why did psychiatry retreat from the care of the developmentally disabled? Our general answer is that psychiatry was ill-prepared to aid in the rehabilitation of these patients. Although much has been learned from investigators with Skinnerian or education-based training, we remain largely ignorant about much of mental retardation. Hence, a central and heartfelt premise in this volume is our conviction that neuropsychiatry has great, albeit unrealized, potential to unravel the mysteries behind understanding and treating the developmentally disabled and their problematic behaviors.

With the advent of new drugs (especially the serotonergic agents) and the routine use of old drugs in new bottles to treat disturbances in behavior, neuropsychiatry is experiencing a dramatic philosophical reorganization. It is a measure of the strength of the humanistic tradition in psychiatry, though, that the field has maintained its essential structures for such a long time, even in the face of the neuropharmacological revolutions. The focus of our therapeutic in-

1

terventions continues to be the interpersonal relationship, the uniqueness of the individual, and his or her refusal to be "lumped" on the basis of an external perspective. These principles are integral to the humanistic point of view.

It is always good to hold on to the worthwhile traditions of the past, but it is sometimes better to take advantage of the opportunities of the present, and it is not always possible to do both at once. The weakness of traditional psychiatry is its failure to accommodate itself, intellectually, to the full impact of the neuropharmacological revolution. We are using the technology, but we are only beginning to create a framework to understand it.

The intellectual division between psychiatrists who emphasize the importance of interpersonal processes and intrapersonal dynamics and psychiatrists who emphasize the importance of common categories and dynamic groups has been a source of tension within the field for about 10 years, and it is still not entirely resolved. In fact, it is our hypothesis, and the working hypothesis of many of the authors in this volume, that this division is a false and unnecessary tension that will never be resolved and masks the real issue that is coming to the fore.

The categories that we must develop are not phenomenological constructs borrowed from old German psychiatrists. The dynamics that we must develop are not the philosophical constructs borrowed from old German neurologists. Rather, we must take our lead from Freud's "Project for a Scientific Psychology" and develop physiological principles of brain function (Freud 1896). The dynamics that we must develop are the interactions between biological mechanisms and external events.

In this chapter, we first expand on our explanations of why psychiatry moved away from treating the mentally retarded. There were two interdependent reasons for this movement. First, psychiatrists were unable to achieve success by grounding their work on a narrow view of the medical model. Second, there was the necessary yet painful intrusion of the legal system into the care of the developmentally disabled. Next, we continue with a thumbnail description of the "new age" in neuropsychiatry—one in which there is a novel, multisystems approach to looking at a patient, an approach that welcomes the contributions of neuropsychiatrists, behaviorists, educators, and others.

PSYCHIATRY'S RETREAT FROM TREATING THE DEVELOPMENTALLY DISABLED

Medical Model

In the "old age" there was the Newtonian medical model—one

genetic defect, one biological abnormality, one cure, with linear causal relationships connecting the links to each other. This Newtonian model of cause and effect is, in essence, a constricted medical model, and it became the psychiatric model propelled by our wish to appear more medical, more scientific, and more respectable. The influence of the medical model, among other things, made possible the popularity of neuroleptic treatment of the developmentally disabled. Further, the widespread use of neuroleptics made possible the profoundly tragic dysfunction of tardive dyskinesia (TD). Finally, public attention to TD facilitated the advent of legal intrusions and substantially contributed to the demoralization of psychiatrists.

Physicians relied on assumptions inherent in the single-cause model for their attempts to find cures for various diseases, such as sickle-cell anemia. Similar assumptions also underlie the rationale behind the dopamine hypothesis of schizophrenia. To describe the characteristics of this approach, however, we illustrate it in terms of one of its most successful progenies—the discovery of a treatment for phenylke-tonuria (PKU), a severe form of mental retardation occurring in approximately 1 of every 15,000 children born in the United States. Researchers found that the early introduction of a phenylalanine-free diet minimized or even eliminated the severity of the dysfunction caused by PKU. Furthermore, researchers determined that PKU was produced by a single recessive gene. Thus, there was only one gene seen as responsible for the development of PKU. This one gene was shown to cause a disturbance in the body's ability to properly metab-olize one amino acid. To prevent this from occurring, only one cure was required—phenylalanine deprivation (Modell 1988).

The assumption in the case of PKU was that if one corrected the overabundance of the PKU amino acid, then the syndrome would be prevented from developing. The error in this assumption lies not within PKU but without it. Psychiatrists, without warrant, took the model for PKU treatment and generalized it to all of psychiatry. For every psychiatric disorder, there became one defect, one drug, one explanation, and one treatment.

Neuroleptic Treatment and Its Forensic Consequences

Psychiatrists became wedded to a deceptively simplistic and reduc-tionist framework: one behavior, one drug. This process gave hope to the more general goal of "medicalizing" psychiatry. Researchers searched for specific actors, specific neurotransmitter sites in the brain, and specific treatments for neuroelectrical abnormalities. Psychiatrists came to see the disorganized thinking pattern of mentally retarded individuals in this same light, as a single disorder with a single treatment. Most notable, the bizarre disruptive behavior of the mentally retarded was regarded as resembling the psychotic behavior associated with schizophrenia.

Neuroleptics were the most effective treatment for psychotic behavior in persons with schizophrenia. If one assumes that one symptom can be alleviated by one drug and that the disruptive behavior of a mentally retarded individual is functionally synonymous with the psychotic behavior of a schizophrenic individual, then one would logically conclude that neuroleptics would be effective in developmentally disabled populations. This, in short, was the inference that many in psychiatry made. As such, the use of neuroleptics was generalized to treat disturbances of any type of severe nonnormal behavior. Eventually, these agents came into vogue as the preferred pharmacological intervention in cases of mental retardation. As C. Thomas Gualtieri writes in Chapter 3 (on the tardive monitoring system), neuroleptics became the "only psychoactive drugs prescribed to mentally retarded people."

Unfortunately, the reasoning that lay behind neuroleptic treatment of developmental disabilities was simplistic, static, and incorrect. Psychiatrists failed to note the long-term consequences of neuroleptic treatment. The catastrophic dysfunction TD later came to the attention of psychiatrists; however, it came to the attention of lawyers as well. The forensic consequences of neuroleptic treatment hastened the departure of psychiatrists from mental retardation in at least two ways. First, public criticism of psychiatrists precipitated a further decline in job satisfaction. Second, the burden of documentation from the intrusion of the legal system became a further aversive condition that made many psychiatrists stop treating developmentally disabled patients.

The movement of the court system into psychiatry has not been gentle in matters dealing with the developmentally disabled. It has been more like a steamroller. The lawsuits, consent decrees, and other forms of legal strictures have led to the reasonable demand that psychopharmacological interventions be carefully scrutinized, documented, and scrupulously tailored. After awareness of TD, many states passed legislation making it difficult to treat the mentally retarded with neuroleptics.

It is unfortunate that the move against neuroleptic treatment was in large part initiated by the judicial system and community agencies, not by psychiatry. The former groups played prominent roles in the professional shift from warehousing the mentally retarded to developing programs with an eye toward habilitation. In human relations, as in pharmacological treatment, psychiatrists proved unable to secure an acceptable quality of life for mentally retarded patients. Psychiatric and developmentally disabled patients did not have an unbiased, naturalistic voice regarding their affairs. A primary achievement of patient advocacy groups was to provide this needed perspective on mental retardation.

Ascendancy of Learning Theorists

With psychiatrists withdrawing from mental retardation care and research, learning theorists and educational psychologists became prominent. These investigators worked to design practices and develop rational approaches to the therapeutics of behavioral programs. Moreover, the work of psychologists and community workers helped create a system of community-living programs that still persists today.

The fiasco of neuroleptic treatment and the ascendance of learning theorists have led to a preoccupation with objective, behavioral criteria—marking a new method of research in the treatment of the developmentally disabled. Previously, psychoanalysis, which relies on subjective reports and theories of the psyche, was the dominant school of thought. Correctly interpreting subjective or introspective data is often a fruitless and unproductive task, however, particularly in those persons with compromised abstraction abilities. In alerting investigators to the importance of scientific research, the influx of learning theorists into the study of mental retardation was a positive development.

Neuropsychiatry can benefit from a close analysis of the biases of behavioral researchers. First, neuropsychiatry should endorse positivistic emphases on the empirical testing and replication of hypotheses. Second, neuropsychiatry should see the advantages in paying close attention to measurement and to the necessity of carefully making constructs operational. For instance, how can we measure aggression in a scientifically acceptable and useful fashion—a fashion amenable to validation and replication (for an attempt, see Silver and Yudofsky 1987)? Third, the behavioral focus on environmental contingencies should alert neuropsychiatrists to the multiple influences, apart from medication, affecting a patient's psychosocial functioning. This notion will be explored in depth in our discussion of the multisystems approach. Finally, the contemporary neuropsychiatrist should share the behaviorist's insistence on adaptation and rehabilitation, rather than on the elusive quest for a definitive cure.

For researchers interested in the treatment of mentally ill patients, a complete cure of patients' illnesses has been regarded as a plausible goal; however, it is unrealistic to posit that the same status of normalcy can be reached by mentally retarded patients. A goal so lofty as to become implausible appears to be deleterious to advancing the state of both the patient and the profession. As such, our emphasis in treating the developmentally disabled has shifted toward ameliorating symptoms and promoting a higher quality of life for patients. The medications prescribed by neuropsychiatrists have powerful effects that can promote or hinder these goals. By carefully testing various polypharmacological regimens, we are confident that neuro-psychiatrists can make invaluable contributions toward the rehabilitation of developmentally disabled patients.

Conclusion: Mindlessness of the Medical Model

Most of us develop a premature cognitive commitment to an outdated set of categories without realizing the possibility of developing new and better-suited ones. The term *premature cognitive commitment* derives from Langer's (1989) "mindlessness" theory—an appropriate, if severe, tag for the old era in psychiatry. A premature cognitive commitment consists of a strong yet blind attachment to a traditional yet maladaptive method of processing one's environment. Psychiatrists, when faced with impossible, upsetting, and seemingly untreatable situations, tended to borrow from diagnostic categories that appeared to offer hope. Recall that the neuroleptics achieved an influential position in the treatment of the mentally retarded largely because they proved successful in treatment of the mentally ill. Therefore, we generalized the medical model from the mentally ill to the mentally retarded. We generalized neuroleptic treatment from the schizophrenic patient to the developmentally disabled individual. Psychiatrists took refuge in diagnostic categories and regarded them as gospel, despite the fact that the diagnostic taxonomy is ever changing and tenuous at best—designed to be a guide, not an absolute, to clinicians. Such generalizations, we see in retrospect, were premature, mindless, and most certainly harmful to the quality of life of the developmentally disabled.

Psychopharmacological treatment goals most often focused on one symptom, behavioral control. Little attention was given to the effects of medications on patients' cognitive or social abilities. Further, we convinced ourselves that we were performing at an optimal level, given limited understanding of the phenomena and an impoverished treatment arsenal. It is now essential to be mindful of patients and to examine the entire spectrum of potential influences, as opposed to maintaining a sole fixation on symptomatology. The negative short- and long-term consequences of pharmacological treatment must be a primary consideration of neuropsychiatrists. Our hope for the future is that improved methods of research will aid neuropsychiatry in determining the various influences that treatment programs may have on patients' well-being.

THE NEW AGE IN NEUROPSYCHIATRY

We have spent a good deal of print lamenting past misfortunes in psychiatry. It has finally become obvious to us that the Newtonian construct has not only failed to advance a patient's quality of life but, indeed, has been deleterious to it. The task of today's neuropsychiatrist is to devise frameworks demonstrating the effectiveness of neuropsychiatry to combat mental illness. And achievement of this state facilitates satisfaction of our goal—to raise the quality of life of the developmentally disabled significantly and dramatically.

Most psychiatrists would consider it presumptuous to say that major changes in the field will come from a field of encephalopathies that is static. It is a field for educators and behaviorists, not physicians. The only valid study in the field is prevention, and the only important physicians working in the field are geneticists. The only role psychiatrists ever had to play was in the bad old days, when they ran the big old state hospitals and training schools. Now they have no role at all. Nothing could be further from the truth.

The study of mental retardation is probably the most fertile intellectual area in the new psychiatry. It is a generation ahead, and the gap is widening. One may hold to the traditional view, that the essence of psychiatry is the diagnosis and treatment of patients with functional or emotional disorders, that psychiatry begins with depression and ends with schizophrenia, and that there is no psychiatric examination if the patient cannot talk. There is always a point to be made, in support of the traditional view. But it is sometimes better to take advantage of new opportunities.

Here are four opportunities for psychiatry in the study of mental retardation:

1. The organization of the field revolves around consumer activism, the primacy of the client, and the responsible development of necessary resources for habilitation and long-term care. The political organization of the field has been led by the families of retarded people for 40 years, and for that reason it has been successful. The political organization of the families of the mentally ill is, by comparison, very new.
2. The treatment of mentally retarded people is not based on unitary disease models; nor is it concentrated in the hands of a few highly

paid professionals, whose services are available to the very few. The essence of treatment is active programming, an ecological approach to the day-to-day and hour-to-hour requirements of the retarded person. When one compares the habilitative programming at a mental-retardation facility with the therapeutic milieu of a psychiatric hospital, the differences are stark.

3. The molecular analysis of behavior and the scientific design of specific behavioral interventions have achieved high levels in mental-retardation facilities. This achievement has lent to the field a positivistic emphasis on the empirical testing and replication of hypotheses. It has lent close attention to careful measurement of behavior and the necessity of carefully making constructs operational. The behavioral focus on environmental contingencies recognizes the importance of multiple influences, apart from the purely biological, that influence a patient's state of mind. And the emphasis of the behaviorist is more appropriately in the direction of adaptation and habilitation, rather than the elusive quest for a definitive cure.

4. On the medical side, the activity of medical geneticists and neurobiologists is indeed remarkable, but it is not oriented exclusively toward prevention. It is also oriented toward the elaboration of specific genetic and biochemical mechanisms that underlie human behavior. Because so many of the syndromes of the developmentally disabled are characterized by stereotypical pathological behavior, an extraordinary opportunity is available to students of brain-behavior relationships.

The chapters of this volume illustrate empirical research founded on a multisystems approach to treatment of the developmentally disabled. In the multisystems approach, the brain and the person are considered a total system, not merely as receptacles for discrete and localized functioning units. Adherents to this view emphasize the external influences impinging on the brain and consider the usefulness of drug regimens that now go beyond preferred categories of the medical model. First, we give an illustration of this approach by briefly discussing the interdependent concepts of noise (Sands and Ratey 1986), psychological trauma (van der Kolk and Greenberg 1987), and kindling (Post and Kopanda 1976; Post et al. 1981). Then, we remark on avenues for treatment and how neuropsychiatrists must emphasize the interconnectedness of behavioral and pharmacological techniques. Finally, we expand on what it means to practice multisystems psychopharmacology and argue that this approach yields the greatest degree of life enhancement to those suffering from developmental disabilities.

Noise

One must be attuned to patients' interactions with the environment and to their history and present state. Neuropsychiatrists should note, for instance, that the developmentally disabled are often vulnerable to traumatic events, or events experienced as traumatic, because of their inability to filter out internal and external stimuli. This dysfunction often occurs because of a misrepresentation of information and subsequent baseline exaggeration of preexisting maladaptive behavior (Sovner 1986). This distortion and hypersensitivity to information may prevent the attainment of normal attention spans.

We have considered this topic at length in our discussions of the *noise* construct (Sands and Ratey 1986). Consider that, just as in a radio wave, the stimuli that all of us receive from the environment are composed partially of signal, useful information, and partially of noise, useless information. The developmentally disabled, we have postulated, process information with, in essence, a low signal-to-noise ratio. Hence, they receive a less-clear signal from stimuli than do able subjects. Conversely, the developmentally disabled receive more noise and clutter than do able subjects.

What behaviors might be observed in able individuals who experience only static in a radio reception or distracting clatter in their conversations? Or in subjects who are subjected to one channel of distracting information in a dichotic listening task? One would be likely to see signs of annoyance, frustration, and irritability. Now picture individuals with a dysfunction making them unable to process information without large proportions of concurrent noise mutating the signal. The attention deficit of schizophrenia, for instance, may be caused by malfunctioning of the selective filter preventing irrelevant stimuli from overwhelming cognition (Maher 1966; Rappaport 1968; Schakow 1950, 1962). This may be conceptualized in terms of the large proportion of noise in information received by a patient.

Psychological Trauma

What may result from experiencing a signal that can be neither integrated nor controlled? Stimulus overload can produce, among other things, internal chaos, personal distortions, impulsivity, hypervigilance, greatly increased physiological stress, and aggression (Glass and Singer 1972; Miller 1959; Sands and Ratey 1986). When the input one receives, from the body and from the external environment, is chaotic and uncontrollable for long periods of time, one tends to respond rigidly in an attempt to organize the stimuli (Goldstein 1948). Other authors have described the drive that patients with schizophrenia (Arieti 1974), delusional patients (Maher 1988), hyperaroused individuals (Festinger 1954; Schachter 1959), and others have to label and otherwise understand their own experiences. These goals are extremely difficult to achieve when perceptual processes fail to mirror events in the world sufficiently. The failure of patients to cope adequately with their unselective filter may result in the onset of helplessness and depression (Seligman 1978).

It should come as no surprise, then, that the inability of some patients to order their experiences is conducive to the trauma response described by van der Kolk and Greenberg (1987). They noted:

> The central nervous system seems to react to any overwhelming threatening and uncontrollable experience in a consistent pattern. Regardless of the precipitating event, traumatized people continue to have a poor tolerance for arousal. They tend to respond to stress in an all-or-nothing way: either unmodulated anxiety, often accompanied by motoric discharge that includes acts of aggression against the self and others, or else social and emotional withdrawal. (Krystal 1978, p. 64)

We postulate that the frequency and intensity of traumatic events are much greater in patients receiving information with a high degree of noise already in place. Hypersensitivity to arousal is particularly acute in the developmentally disabled, because incoming arousal stimuli may already be experienced as exaggerated beyond their initial magnitude. Further, the increased arousal characteristic of traumatized individuals, even if not initially distorted as in the developmentally disabled, becomes a precipitant to and not a preparation for dangerous scenarios. This also weakens the correlation between the amount of anxiety felt and the anxiety required to adaptively respond to environmental stressors.

Kindling Hypothesis

The hyperarousal felt by many developmentally disabled patients has a spiraling effect. The exaggeration of incoming stimuli facilitates a state of increased sensitivity to further stimuli and relatively chronic traumatization. The trauma, in turn, heightens the amount of arousal felt in the environment, above and beyond the misinterpretation of stimuli caused by the inability to censor irrelevant stimuli. The spiraling structure captured here is better described by use of Post's kindling hypothesis (Post and Kopanda 1976; Post et al. 1981). Kindling was first discovered as a bioelectrical phenomenon by Goddard et al. (1969), when they noted that the repeated yet intermittent excitation of a brain site with subthreshold currents may eventually produce major motor seizures in an individual. Post indicated that similar consequences may ensue from psychosocial, not just electrical, stressors; even if initially trivial they may, if repeated long enough, foster the onset of severe behavioral disturbances. Developmentally disabled patients may suffer from distorted and chaotic stimuli, which in isolation are not capable of promoting dysfunction but over time lead to tragic disturbances. Repeated activation of neural pathways by stressors may actually change the biochemistry of the brain.

The multisystems approach stresses the interdependencies of behavior and biology and the necessity of understanding both to attain an adequate understanding of developmental disabilities. The theories of noise, trauma, and kindling present a relatively coherent, if threatening, picture of an infant born with a developmental disability. Noise processed by the infant may eventually, through the kindling mechanism, produce profound and terrorizing psychological trauma. As van der Kolk and Greenberg (1987) pointed out, the uncontrolled nature of the noisy stimuli makes a traumatic response more likely. Initial subthreshold neuronal excitation precipitated by frustration, hypervigilance, impulsivity, and the like may sensitize these pathways to further activation. Not only does tolerance of noise fail to develop, the chronicity of this dysfunction may make severe disturbances much more likely in the future. Environmental effects can produce actual changes in the physiology of the brain. Moreover, these biological changes facilitate further developmental decay, contributing to the pathology of the developmentally disabled.

Multisystems Approach and Its Concern
for Patients' Quality of Life

How can we treat patients suffering from disabilities such as high noise levels in stimuli? In a broad sense, we must use a more holistic perspective toward mental retardation. Ideally, psychiatrists employ medications to improve the functioning of mentally retarded patients. The departure of psychiatrists and the subsequent ascendancy of behaviorists in the treatment of the developmentally disabled has artificially widened the conceptual gap between neuropsychiatrists and behaviorists. With the multisystems approach, we consider the behavior and the biology as complementary and not antagonistic aspects of the person requiring treatment. (Such a treatment does not seem revolutionary until one examines the history of our field.) Like the past contingencies of the environment, pharmacological interventions determine behavior; indeed, they are internal controllers of behavior. Considering the task before us, it is essential to use the full knowledge of both the neuropsychiatric and the behavior theory researchers in the new age of psychiatry.

Therefore, we not only pay closer attention to the external environment in the multisystems approach, we also must be attuned to the pharmacological environment. Drugs may modify the microenvironment in the specific synaptic neighborhood of the brain rather than have a pure antagonistic effect. Presently in neuropsychiatry, we see a burgeoning of nontraditional treatments for behavioral problems. By nontraditional we mean that these pharmacotherapies not only cut across the overcodified *Diagnostic and Statistical Manual of Mental Disorders* diagnostic categories but also increase our understanding of behavior. A neuropsychiatrist attuned to the multisystems approach may be less likely to err toward the deceptively simplistic one-drug, one-symptom model and thus may be more likely to contribute to the general life enhancement of a patient.

Throughout this chapter, we have placed a strong emphasis on improving the quality of life of the developmentally disabled. Psychiatrists, we have suggested, are better served by attempting to rehabilitate a patient than by searching for definitive interventions that can effectively eliminate the behavioral problems associated with mental retardation or by employing medications merely for the purposes of sedation. In large part, the present program is a reaction against previous psychiatric practices. In the past, the drug regimens administered to patients often culminated in side effects ranging from impaired cognitive functioning to the onset of TD. In this chapter, we have discussed in detail the ramifications of this malfeasance for the developmentally disabled and their clinicians.

What measures can be taken to improve the quality of life for psychiatric patients? How are we to go about implementing a program of rehabilitation? As a point of departure, we would be well advised to consider the vantage point of Mandell (1986). In writing about the challenge of psychopharmacology, Mandell noted:

> Subtle clinical observation seldom is allowed to expand the vistas of the model builders and the drug developers. . . . The best psychopharmacologists managing severely ill patients use several, unusual, and often (theoretically) antagonistic drugs carefully tailored over many months of adjustment to minimize side-effects and maximize desired effect. (p. 362)

Within this excerpt are several guidelines worthy of expansion. Foremost is the need "to minimize side-effects and maximize desired effect." To minimize side effects, we must realize the necessity of searching for less-toxic medications. Concurrent with this is the attractiveness of maximizing desired effects, to target drugs therapeutically for individual patients.

Mandell (1986) wrote that optimal treatment programs 1) may be multipharmic, 2) may employ doses considered homeopathic, 3) may be used in conjunction with clinical observations of behavior, and 4) are perfected over time in accord with research and experimentation. Fortunately, the process of developing pharmacotherapies is greatly facilitated by the advent of new medical technologies. These instruments may give neuropsychiatrists great insight into the nature of mental retardation and thus may constitute a powerful impetus for psychiatric research.

The most effective regimen often consists of an intervention employing more than one medication. Needless to say, a polypharmacological approach is unnecessary given a conceptual model in which one symptom is alleviated by one drug. If, however, the dysfunctions of developmentally disabled patients are conceptualized as products of a dynamic causal network, or (as Post would have it) a negative spiral, then the use of more than one medication at a time should be given close attention by a clinician.

Possible interventions, whether consisting of one or several drugs, should be tested despite a priori notions of ineffectiveness. Neuropsychiatrists are realizing that drugs previously believed to have no bearing on psychiatric symptoms often convey positive effects. Medications commonly used in internal medicine—such as amantadine, naltrexone, the anticonvulsants, and the β-blockers—are all prominently featured in this book. As we have noted throughout our chapter, the preconceived constructs of psychiatrists have often led us to ignore behavioral syndromes and potential treatment programs. For example, Frank Menolascino, Stephen Ruedrich and Jasbir Kang, in Chapter 2, write of how psychiatrists have been trapped by their own stereotypes of such dysfunctions as Down's syndrome. We have not, in Mandell's (1986) words addressing psychiatry as a whole, been "creative" in devising pharmacotherapies successful in rehabilitation. Considering how little we really know about the pharmacology of mental retardation, it is foolhardy to reject the use of a host of psychopharmacological interventions without prior testing.

Mandell's (1986) emphasis on "subtle clinical observation" implies that neuropsychiatrists should pay more attention to the objective manifestations of behavior. Pharmacotherapies should be integrated with behavioral techniques and behavioral programs. In treatment of panic or a depressive episode, for example, minute doses of psychoactive drugs may lead to a near-complete change in the behavioral and social capabilities of a developmentally disabled patient. With judicious use of medications, patients may become useful players, not disruptions, in a ward.

Neuropsychiatrists must hone their ability to help the developmentally disabled through the force of their ideas and objective standards of evidence, not through a blind application of the "right" treatment for the "right" symptom. And ideas, as Mandell (1986) argued, should be subjected to empirical tests. In the process of hypothesis formation and testing, theories simultaneously grow and become more refined, to a point where, one hopes, rational regimens and expectations are met and then applied to other areas.

The generation and testing of hypotheses will be a hallmark of the new age in neuropsychiatry. Further, empirical research will be much helped by another new age in science—the new age in technology. Recent advances in neuropsychiatry and medical technology make implementation of the multisystems approach more fruitful, exciting, and informative. The use of new technology for the benefit of the developmentally disabled allows us to understand better the multiple forces impinging on psychiatric patients. Autism, for example, can now be examined on MRI and positron-emission tomography scans to determine neuroanatomical abnormalities in living patients. The developmentally disabled have been a testing ground of the latest generation of medical equipment. Not only is the one-symptom, one-drug model conceptually inefficacious; now, with the penetration of new technology into our laboratories, the medical model is no longer even a metaphorical simplification worth keeping. Bauman's work, for instance, has used a computer-assisted postmortem study that has led to the identification of various brain abnormalities (Bauman and Kemper 1985). This allows us not only to further our understanding of behavior but also to generate hypotheses for treatment.

Many of the contributors to this book offer their hypotheses and their data concerning the development of more-efficacious, less-toxic regimens. John Ratey's chapter with Karen Lindem (Chapter 4), on the peripheral β-blockers, illustrates how the noise level in a patient's awareness can be reduced, and the probability of trauma diminished, without conveying severe side effects to the patient. Unlike centrally acting β-blockers (e.g., propranolol), peripherally acting β-blockers (e.g., nadolol) do not pass the blood-brain barrier. Nonetheless, nadolol has impressive anxiety-relieving and antiaggressive properties. We have thus hypothesized that at least a part of the antiaggressive action of the β-blockers is attained by relaxing the skeletal and striate musculature. This seems to allow a decrease in the bodily contribution to the noise level and a concurrent increase in the patient's subjective feeling of organization, disrupting the catastrophic kindling cycle. Indeed, it may even institute a positive spiral.

In Chapter 2, Frank Menolascino, Jasbir Kang, and Stephen Ruedrich comment on how new developments in neuropsychiatry may foster the general life enhancement of mentally retarded individuals who are also mentally ill. They caution the forthcoming generation of neuropsychiatrists—imploring them to piece apart symptomatology, to consider the entire range of behaviors, and to avoid incorrect and inappropriate stereotypes.

Barbara Herman's chapter (Chapter 6) on the opiate antagonists adds another area of concern and possible avenues of treatment to enhance the quality of life of patients heretofore considered untreatable. As she writes, the opiate antagonists do not affect cognitive structures, allowing patients to be more amenable to behavioral treatment programs.

In Chapter 7, Mark Chandler, L. Jarrett Barnhill, and C. Thomas Gualtieri write of the potential use of amantadine for a population of patients who have not been helped by past pharmacological interventions. Developmentally disabled patients who receive either little pharmacological treatment or treatments with poor toxicity profiles may enjoy great benefits from a drug regimen that includes amantadine.

Robert Sovner (Chapter 5) argues that anticonvulsants—such as carbamazepine, clonazepam, and valproate—should be the medications of first choice when treating affective disorders or organic brain syndromes in mentally retarded patients. He provides a literature review of anticonvulsant use and concludes that they are less toxic, yet more efficacious, than lithium, antipsychotics, or antidepressants.

The propensity of drugs to disturb the microenvironment of the synaptic space may prove to be the most essential feature of the drug-treatment profile. In Chapter 3, C. Thomas Gualtieri discusses how one forms a reasonable regimen for developmentally disabled patients suffering from neuroleptic addiction. The tardive monitoring system (TMS) is developed to aid clinicians composing a suitable mixture of drugs specific to each patient unable to withdraw completely from past neuroleptic treatment. Hence, the TMS is a system for prevention and control of TD and the other tragic effects of neuroleptic use.

The pharmacotherapies discussed by this book's contributors share the concerns of the multisystems approach. Not only are these drugs relatively nontoxic to the brain, they may even confer a cognitively enhancing effect on patients. As a unit, the chapters in this book contain some of the first fruits of the methodology of hypothesis generation and testing, and the paradigm of the multisystem, in the new age in neuropsychiatry.

REFERENCES

Arieti S: Interpretation of Schizophrenia, 2nd Edition. New York, Basic Books, 1974

Bauman M, Kemper TL: Histoanatomic observations of the brain in early autism. Neurology 35:866–874, 1985

Festinger L: A theory of social comparison processes. Human Relations 7:114–140, 1954

Freud S: The aetiology of hysteria (1896), in The Standard Edition of the Complete Psychological Works of Sigmund Freud, Vol 3. Translated and edited by Strachey J. London, Hogarth Press, 1954, pp 178–229

Glass GV, Singer JE: Urban Stress: Experiments on Noise and Social Stressors. New York, Academic, 1972

Goddard GV, McIntyre DC, Leech CK: A permanent change in brain function resulting from daily electrical stimulations. Exp Neurol 25:295–330, 1969

Goldstein K: After Effects of Brain Injuries in War. New York, Grune & Stratton, 1948

Krystal H: Trauma and affects. Psychoanal Study Child 33:81–116, 1978

Langer EJ: Mindfulness. New York, Addison-Wesley, 1989

Maher BA: Principles of Psychopathology. New York, McGraw-Hill, 1966

Maher BA: Anomolous experience and delusional thinking: the logic of explanations, in Delusional Beliefs. Edited by Otmanns TF, Maher BA. New York, John Wiley, 1988, pp 176–219

Mandell AJ: From molecular biological simplification to more realistic central nervous system dynamics: an opinion, in Psychiatry: Psychobiological Foundations of Clinical Psychiatry, Vol 4. Edited by Judd J, Grove P. New York, Basic Books, 1986, pp 361–366

Miller JG: Information overload and psychopathology. Am J Psychother 133:627–634, 1959

Modell B: Distribution and control of some genetic disorders. World Health Stat Q 41(3-4):209–218, 1988

Post RM, Kopanda RT: Cocaine, kindling and psychosis. Am J Psychiatry 133:627–634, 1976

Post RM, Ballenger JC, Uhde TW, et al: Kindling and drug sensation: implications for the progressive development of psychopathology and treatment with carbamazepine, in The Psychopharmacology of Anticonvulsants. Edited by Sanler M. New York, Oxford University Press, 1981, pp 27–53

Rappaport M: Attention to competing voice messages by nonacute schizophrenic patients: effects of message load, drugs, dosage levels and patient background. J Nerv Ment Dis 146:404–411, 1968

Sands S, Ratey J: The concept of noise. Psychiatry 49:290–297, 1986

Schachter S: The Psychology of Affiliation. Stanford, CA, Stanford University Press, 1959

Shakow D: Some psychological features of schizophrenia, in Feelings and Emotions. Edited by Reymart ML. New York, McGraw-Hill, 1950, pp 79–107

Schakow D: Segmental set: a theory of the formal psychological deficit in schizophrenia. Arch Gen Psychiatry 6:1–17, 1962

Seligman ME: Learned helplessness as a model of depression: comment and integration. J Abnorm Psychol 87(1):167–179, 1978

Silver JM, Yudofsky SC: Documentation of aggression in the assessment of the violent patient. Psychiatric Annals 176:375–384, 1987

Sovner R: Limiting factors in the use of DSM-III criteria with mentally ill/mentally retarded persons. Psychopharmacol Bull 22:1055–1059, 1986

van der Kolk BA, Greenberg MS: The psychobiology of the trauma response: hyperarousal, constriction and addiction to traumatic response, in Psychological Trauma. Edited by van der Kolk BA. Washington, DC, American Psychiatric Press, 1987, pp 63–87

Chapter 2

Mental Illness in the Mentally Retarded: Diagnostic Clarity as a Prelude to Psychopharmacological Interventions

Frank J. Menolascino, M.D., Stephen L. Ruedrich, M.D., and Jasbir S. Kang, M.D.

A mental illness that occurs in conjunction with mental retardation poses major diagnostic difficulties and intriguing treatment challenges. The differential diagnostic issues involved in separating the social-adaptive behavioral indices of a moderately retarded individual from his or her concurrent problems in interpersonal transactions can approach the complexity of the Gordian knot. Yet it is only the clear resolution of such issues that can enhance the probability of making astute selections among an increasing number of treatment options.

It may be prudent at the outset to recall how many of the recent advances in this specialized area of psychopharmacology followed a period during which indiscriminate use of psychotropic agents in these patients was common (Lipton 1970). The sedative role of psychotropic medications, by virtue of excessive dosages, was stressed as a thin rationalization for "keeping the patient quiet," which was presumed to be better than providing no treatment. Yet this "something" versus "nothing" approach fostered potentially harmful and restrictive practices. More bluntly, much of this early clinical psychopharmacology represented a nonpsychiatric approach, wherein the control of behavior was exclusively emphasized. Treatment guidelines based on the careful descriptive psychiatric study of an individualized clinical picture failed to be considered. Sovner (1986) and others (Aman 1985; Aman and Singh 1986; Colodny and Kurlander 1970; Stark et al. 1984) have, in a series of incisive papers, documented this period of dark clinical intervention, during which the quelling of behavioral turmoil was viewed as the primary goal. Such was the ethos of treatment nihilism that pervaded the field of mental retardation before and during the 1950s and 1960s.

The past two decades have taken a fresh appraisal of the psychiatric aspects of mental retardation (Menolascino 1970), wherein the DSM-III (American Psychiatric Association 1980) and more recently the DSM-III-R (American Psychiatric Association 1987) diagnostic systems began to be applied to the behavioral syndromes noted in the mentally retarded. Modern training approaches are being increasingly embraced, and guidelines for most modern psychiatric treatment interventions on behalf of the dually diagnosed are being explored (American Psychiatric Association 1989; Fletcher and Menolascino, in press; McGee and Pearson 1983; Stark and Menolascino 1986). It is against this bright backdrop of recent progress that the context of this book can promise such exciting possibilities in terms of effective psychopharmacological intervention for our mentally retarded and mentally ill citizens.

PSYCHIATRIC ASSESSMENT OF BEHAVIORAL DISTURBANCE IN THE MENTALLY RETARDED: OBJECTIVE BEHAVIORAL ASSESSMENT

The literature in mental-health and mental-retardation research reveals a growing professional focus on descriptive diagnosis and on the objectively delineated phenomena that are clinically present, instead of possible causative mechanisms or indirect dynamic formulations so typical of the recent past. For example, many professional myths regarding the expected behavioral symptoms of mentally retarded citizens have led to stilted diagnostic approaches that tend to dismiss the efficacy of psychiatric treatment interventions and disallow hopeful prognoses. Many health care professionals were trained to believe (or had fixed personal views before ever starting advanced training) that, in contrast to normal persons, mentally retarded citizens display qualitative or quantitative distinctiveness in their expressions of the signs and symptoms of mental illness. A clear instance of this excessive concentration on extraneous factors was the commonly held assumption that individuals with Down's syndrome were the "Prince Charmings" of the mentally retarded: overly friendly, extremely affable, given to mimicry, and devoid of personality conflicts. Unfortunately, this particular behavioral stereotype blinded generations of clinicians to the wide spectrum of abnormal behaviors that Down's syndrome patients presented directly before their eyes, causing them to concentrate instead on the traditional interpretations of anticipated behaviors. As the psychiatric dimensions of Down's syndrome began to be studied and reported in the literature, however, the Prince Charming facade fell away, revealing a wide array of psychiatric disorders (Lund 1988; Lund and Munk-Jorgenson 1988; Stark et al. 1988).

Progress is being made, therefore, in that the measurement and recording of atypical or abnormal behaviors via descriptive scales, some of which have greater validity than others, are increasingly replacing the hypothesized presence of signs or symptoms of mental illness in the mentally retarded (Matson 1988; Reiss et al. 1982; Sonnander 1986; Watson et al. 1988). Clinicians seem less comfortable viewing and describing *multiple* symptomatic/syndromic phenomena and acting directly on them through multiple treatment interventions. Instead, they tend to follow the traditional training principle of seeking the major cause of given symptom configurations and then using the rather myopic treatment procedures that flow from such a one-dimensional (and most often erroneous) approach. Admittedly, the challenge of diagnosing a mentally retarded or mentally ill person, who may well display from six to eight major presenting symptoms, tends to bewilder clinicians. It is becoming increasingly clear, however, that the evolving postures of descriptive diagnostic clarification as a prelude to specific treatment intervention will continue to help erase the aura of bewilderment that has clouded the vision of mental-health professionals toward dually diagnosed persons in the past.

A particularly strong antidote to any ongoing overreliance on behavioral stereotypes in the mentally retarded is the multidisciplinary team approach with its more balanced strategies for diagnosis and treatment interventions. Such an approach, which brings together a wide range of talents and skills in an effort to clarify these complex clinical challenges, entails an attendant professional posture wherein a premium is placed on the clear description of current behaviors. One can only treat what is present, whether in mentally retarded mentally ill patients or in nonretarded mentally ill patients. True, a psychoanalyst might scoff at such a simplistic view of human behavior, but he or she would have to concede that it is behavioral improvement that most conflicted or mentally retarded persons are requesting of our clinical intervention efforts and that the psychoanalytical goal of reeducation of the personality is now viewed as a rare luxury, both in its attainment and in terms of patient (or parental/caretaker) interest. In other words, most people want to obtain prompt relief for their headaches (disturbing feelings) and are not overly interested in knowing the symbolic basis for them.

The use of a wide variety of direct treatment approaches for objectively described behaviors has been a hallmark of developmentally oriented treatment-management approaches in the field of mental retardation for more than two decades. It is now, and will increasingly be, more actively extended into the arena of clinical management of the mental illnesses that are so commonly noted in this population.

PRIMITIVE, ATYPICAL, AND ABNORMAL BEHAVIOR IN THE MENTALLY RETARDED

Whether psychopharmacology is considered a primary or secondary treatment intervention in the mentally retarded, it is important to separate out that wide etiological spectrum in which developmental or psychosocial aspects of the symptom of mental retardation distinctly color the clinical presentation. Herein the behavioral accompaniments of primitive, atypical, and abnormal behaviors can help to clarify for a clinician just what does (and does not) warrant active treatment. This diagnostic dimension is especially important when one notes that many instances of self-injurious or noncompliant behavior in the mentally retarded are reflections of delayed development rather than psychopathology.

Primitive Behavior

Primitive behavior is usually manifested by severely or profoundly retarded individuals who additionally display gross delays in their language development. The primitive behaviors most consistently displayed stem from the extremely limited behavioral repertoires so often noted in these patients, particularly within the context of excessive expectations from their families, their educational milieu, their group home staff, a vocational training setting, and so forth. Such behaviors involve rudimentary use of special sensory modalities, particularly touch, position, oral exploratory activity, and sudden verbalizations that have no apparent purpose in terms of interpersonal communication. In diagnostic interviews, primitive behaviors—such as the mouthing and licking of objects, excessive tactile stimulation, autistic hand movements, skin picking, and body rocking—are frequently noted. In severely retarded children, the very primitiveness of their overall behavior, in conjunction with much stereotyping, may initially suggest a psychotic disorder of childhood. Such youngsters will, however, slowly make sustained eye contact and interact with their examiners if carefully and indirectly approached, despite their minimal behavioral repertoires. Similarly, one might form the initial impression that the level and persistence of primitive behaviors are actually secondary to intrinsic or extrinsic deprivation factors. Yet on further investigation, these children clearly display concurrent multiple indices of developmental arrest of either primary or congenital origin. Clarifying the diagnosis, realigning parental and professional expectations, and focusing on specific developmental and educational transactional modalities are the keys to providing effective help to mentally retarded individuals who display these primitive behaviors.

It is within this framework of a primitive behavioral picture that a clinician must determine which dysfunctional behaviors (e.g., impulsiveness, hyperactivity, and shortened attention span) should be treated on a symptomatic basis. The psychopharmacological agents to be used should then be selected in a manner similar to that employed for organic brain syndromes—that is, through matching the pharmacological interventions with the etiologies that produced the symptoms of mental retardation. For example, anticonvulsants may be prescribed for posttraumatic (closed head) injuries that have features of attention-deficit disorders but no allied seizure phenomena. Similarly, in instances that reflect cranial malformations as an underlying etiology, pharmacological agents, such as propranolol, should be considered for their peripheral locus of action in selectively modulating primitive behavioral dysfunctions. Since these and similar psychopharmacological agents are used to alter symptoms selectively, it is imperative that they are always used within the context of a balanced educational, vocational, and social-recreational management program.

Atypical Behavior

Atypical behaviors include poor emotional control (as evidenced by emotional outbursts), impulsiveness, sullenness, obstinacy, mild legal transgressions, and generally poor adaptation to prevocational or vocational training programs. For example, a mentally retarded adolescent may be committed to an institution because of ongoing adjustment difficulties within his or her home community, but it is important to note that such difficulties are not experienced within the primary family structure. Instances of atypical behavior may only be atypical for the institutional settings in which these individuals find themselves, since they are usually quite typical within the subculture of the patients' primary family (i.e., dysocial phenomena). In the *Manual of Terminology and Classification in Mental Retardation* (Grossman 1983), etiologic diagnosis is usually in the realm of cultural-familial or idiopathic mental retardation. When an individual of this type arrives at an institution, psychiatric consultation is most commonly requested because the patient refuses to cooperate with the training or social expectations of the institutional setting or because continual abrasive comments or contact from the family belittles the institution's ability to help the patient. The family may actually deny the reality of any social-adaptive problems or harass the institutional staff for focusing on and attempting to modify problem behaviors. As Beitenman (1981) noted, however, the clarification of both familial expectations and the roles of clinicians and staff members is necessary before these patients can be managed appropriately for all concerned parties.

It would seem that formerly institutionalized mentally retarded individuals with atypical behavior are increasingly "flunking out" of community-based service programs and continue their persistently atypical behavior within a social system other than the primary family. Clinical management of these complex cases is difficult unless close coordination exists between the administrative segments of institutional treatment teams. Nevertheless, during a period of crises, the total environment of an institution can help redirect motivational potential, effect realistic changes in the expectations these individuals have of themselves and others, and assist these individuals in achieving more positive social-adaptive approaches to interpersonal transactions and the world of work.

The cautions previously noted as to when or if to treat primitive behaviors also apply to the atypical behaviors presented by these mentally retarded citizens, who constitute 75% or more of the youngsters (or adults) with pervasive developmental disturbance. Typically, they have a long-standing history of atypical general and behavioral developmental disturbance. These complex individuals can be quite challenging—especially as they grow older (and physically larger)—because their behavioral repertories become increasingly difficult for parents, teachers, and vocational-center helpers to manage. Often, ongoing psychoactive drug management becomes a series of attempts specifically designed to alter restlessness, aggressive propensities, and markedly self-centered or self-abusive behaviors and activities.

To date, however, the available psychopharmacological treatment interventions for these complex individuals tend to be nonspecific and lose their effectiveness within several years' time (Donaldson 1984; Menolascino and McCann 1983). Nevertheless, current research and allied treatment approaches to the more effective management of these types of atypical, self-injurious, and noncompliant behaviors are excellently illustrated in the chapters of this book and hold great promise for more specific and effective intervention in the near future.

Abnormal Behavior: Syndromes of Mental Illness in the Mentally Retarded

A large percentage of the clearly abnormal behavioral challenges encountered in institutionalized or community-based samples of mentally retarded individuals tends to encompass psychotic behaviors. It is truly remarkable that one still sees psychotic patients who have been literally dumped into institutions for the mentally retarded because of the absence of specific treatment programs in their home communities. One typically notes a clinical history of great enthusiasm when treatment is initiated, but slowness of response is often disillusioning, and the patient is referred to another colleague as "nontreatable." A broad view of developmental potentials and psychotic characteristics must be wedded to specific treatment goals if this type of treatment nihilism or failure is to be avoided.

In clinical interviews, young retarded persons with psychotic disorders tend to present the following behavioral dimensions: 1) bizarreness of manner, gesture, and posture; 2) uncommunicative speech; 3) little or no discrimination between animate and inanimate objects; 4) identification with most inanimate objects; 5) deviant affective expression; 6) few, if any, relationships with peers; 7) passive compliance to external demands or stimuli; 8) marked negativism. Many institutions for the mentally retarded have built up large backlogs of psychotic patients whose definitive treatment needs have never been appropriately addressed. Such patients are typically referred elsewhere during acute episodes and returned in subacute remission states. Because institutional staff members frequently view these individuals as odd or dangerous, the psychotic process is often refueled by apprehensive personnel until a patient once again enters an acute stage of chronic mental illness.

Beyond these general considerations are the challenges inherent in attempting to confirm a psychotic disorder in a severely retarded, nonverbal individual. In approaching a final configuration of the indices of mental illness, it is important to remember the wide array of biological markers that have become available in recent years, such as the dexamethasone suppression test in instances of major depression and the lactate infusion assessment for panic disorders. In addition, the new neuroimaging techniques, such as positron-emission tomography (Jacobson 1988; Montgomery 1989), have provided modern psychiatry with one of its first biopsy techniques and hold great promise for objectively assessing the severely retarded, who so often cannot speak well about their turmoil, if they are able to speak at all.

Through the use of DSM-III-R criteria, which arrange mental illness on Axis I and the concurrent presence of mental retardation on Axis II, the old diagnostic merry-go-round (which one came first?) can be more easily avoided. A diagnostic impression can be clearly stated and elaborated in terms of the specific time of developmental onset and the initial behavioral manifestations. For example, the syndrome of pervasive developmental disturbance, the symptoms of which tend to be amenable to psychopharmacological intervention, is now placed on Axis II, and only the acute, superimposed symptoms of concurrent mental illness (e.g., an Axis I major unipolar depression) prompt the need for specific treatment intervention. Indeed, the presence of organic brain syndrome does not mean that dually diagnosed patients are nontreatable, since different treatment interventions are clarified by the Axis I/Axis II entities (e.g., the new DSM-III-R 307.30 stereotypy/habit disorder entity). These considerations call for a closer examination of the bipolar disorders, the masked self-injurious behaviors noted in a wide variety of clinical syndromes, and the transitional adjustment disorders, which, in my experience, have too infrequently been reported in the professional literature. Childhood depression can serve as an analogy here: Until 5 years ago it was considered a rare phenomenon, whereas today it is commonly reported (but still rarely noted in the literature on mental illness in the mentally retarded).

Although it would be easy to state straightforwardly that the specific mental illnesses noted in the retarded should be those syndromes fulfilling DSM-III-R guidelines, it is important to remember that certain symptoms have been *elevated* to a status indicative of mental illness. For example, the descriptors *self-injurious behaviors* and *noncompliant behaviors* are often regarded as diagnostic entities in need of treatment. Yet both descriptors are noted 1) in a high percentage of nonretarded people (especially young people), 2) in schizophrenia, 3) in seizure equivalents, 4) in affective disorders, 5) as a partial symptom of autism, and 6) as volitional behaviors (i.e., a variant of normal behavior or a slowly solidifying character disorder). Rather than engage in arbitrary diagnostic inclusion, it has been my repeated experience that close and prolonged observation always eventuates in a descriptive diagnostic impression. This posture, which I strongly advocate, must include the use of the descriptor *no psychiatric disorder* and the increased use of the relatively benign descriptor *adjustment disorders* with their parameters of crisis and time. Firm adherence to the medical model also helps to clarify those hazy behavioral pictures (i.e., clusters of what appear on initial evaluation to be unrelated descriptive symptoms) so frequently seen in the mentally retarded. These vague *initial* clinical pictures will consistently give way to clear DSM-III-R designations or other challenging entities, such as organic anxiety secondary to hyperthyroidism, vitamin B_{12} deficiency masking as atypical depression, and instances of amphetamine toxicity that look like schizophrenia in the mentally retarded and nonretarded alike. Again, close observation of symptom clusters, especially secondary to supportive (and initially nonspecific) care, will help to clarify diagnostic entities as a prelude to asking whether pharmacotherapy adjuncts are needed.

An Allied Issue: The Most Complex Challenges

Three subgroups of the mentally retarded—severely retarded multiply handicapped persons, mentally retarded mentally ill persons, and mentally retarded persons with criminal proclivities (i.e., mentally retarded "offenders")—also have major behavioral or personality difficulties as core problems. Although the physical needs of severely retarded multiply handicapped persons tend to emanate directly from their extremely delayed and restricted abilities to deal with the external world, their behaviors also have direct repercussions on their families, their caregivers, and society in general. These individuals tend to exhaust their parents physically and emotionally, and they represent a huge dose of reality to overzealous treatment personnel who seem unable to wait for or tolerate the typically slow developmental timetables of these handicapped and complex retarded citizens.

Similar professional challenges surround the issue of providing treatment for a mentally retarded and chronically delinquent adolescent (or offending adult) who displays maladaptive, aggressive, or abnormal sexual proclivities. Indeed, the difficulties involved in providing effective care to this subpopulation are exceptional because the field of corrections (where the bulk of these individuals may belong, rather than in mental-retardation service systems through inappropriate referral) has a much weaker base of professional involvement or ongoing parental support than do the developmental-educational mental-health systems of care. Although this particular subgroup is not large numerically, these individuals do tend to tie up excessive amounts of staff time, and their behavioral volatility is an ever-present disruptive influence in mental-retardation service systems. Although it has become a truism that an adolescent delinquent can and should be treated via the current models of care in adolescent psychiatry (Day 1988), this truism awaits fuller implementation as increasing numbers of mental-health personnel become actively involved. A mentally retarded adult who consistently has legal entanglements secondary to his or her poor impulse control tends to respond to mental-health treatment approaches. For such individuals, the future trend will be to involve them more directly in the correctional system of care while providing active mental-health inputs and mental-retardation services on an ongoing consultation basis.

The future cadres of health care professionals who serve dually diagnosed patients will need more than the one-dimensional training currently characteristic of mental-retardation and mental-health education. Modern training must also focus on the basic concepts and sets of experiences that the various members of an interdisciplinary team will need to be truly able to provide proficient, up-to-date viewpoints and techniques regarding diagnosis and treatment. Such exposure will permit mental-health trainees to understand more readily and appreciate their clinical transactions with mentally retarded patients and their parents. An educated awareness of the unique needs of mentally retarded citizens—regardless of whether they are also mentally ill—will prepare mental health care workers to incorporate those specialized treatment-management techniques that have proven to be consistently helpful to this dually diagnosed population. Experiences derived from both fields of expertise will produce a far more knowledgeable and compassionate mental health care practitioner for whatever population the individual focuses on in his or her future professional career.

GENERAL DIAGNOSTIC CONCERNS

As psychiatry more strongly embraces the biopsychosocial model, it has become increasingly clear that the complexity of the diagnostic entities noted must be matched by equally complex or definitive treatment interventions. Just as the designation *early infantile autism* once occasioned erroneous diagnostic-etiologic considerations and allied treatment approaches, current focus on such issues as the exploration of family histories associated with the affective disorders must now come to be more carefully understood: Is there significant genetic loading? Is psychosocially programmed passivity slowly erupting into manic (motoric) explosion? Is organic personality syndrome (i.e., secondary to tumor, trauma, etc.) masking as a potentially treatable underlying cause? Similarly, the concept of diagnostic overshadowing (Reiss et al. 1982), in which the symptoms of mental illness are overshadowed (in the clinician's mind) by the syndrome of mental retardation, applies to such blind spots. The clinical distortions so often noted in mentally retarded mentally ill patients (e.g., intellectual distortion, psychosocial masking, cognitive disintegration, and baseline exaggeration) can result in the "diagnostic vision problems" so clearly outlined by Sovner (1986, 1988).

Many of the contributors to this book have used the subtleties of behavioral psychopharmacology to examine the empirical treatment approaches that are increasingly being applied (and reported) in the innovative care of dually diagnosed patients. It is important to stress the need for health care professionals to use pharmacological agents (e.g., anticonvulsants) more flexibly as potentially helpful differential diagnostic instruments. The principle here is atypically traditional in that a closely monitored response to medication is viewed as being potentially therapeutically helpful and clarifying in terms of concomitant diagnostic challenges. This approach becomes even more viable, in my opinion, when working with dually diagnosed patients because of their multiple etiologies and need for balanced treatment approaches and flexibility in treatment trials. These complex mentally retarded citizens truly require remediation over time, not the "quick fix" of crisis-to-crisis pharmacological intervention. Debates regarding the merits of short- and long-term treatment approaches highlight certain associated dangers, such as incorrect diagnoses, poor monitoring of treatment, and the need for timely intervention. As mentally retarded mentally ill patients are cared for over time, clinicians tend to use psychopharmacological adjuncts less and less as a primary treatment intervention (except in clear-cut disorders, such as acute episodes of schizophrenia). Instead, clinicians increasingly rely on psychosocial and educational-vocational approaches to long-term personality changes.

As we continue to try to understand more fully the nature of mental illness in mentally retarded individuals, it becomes clear that we need to reexamine the more frequently reported mental illnesses in non-retarded individuals (e.g., reactive psychosis, the adjustment disorders, and crisis situations) and to question why these illnesses are so rarely reported in the mentally retarded population. The reality-based difficulties, for which mentally retarded mentally ill individuals are always more at risk, present us with a continuous professional challenge that we have as complete a grasp on the existential setting of these individuals as possible (Ghaziuddin 1988). For example, de-institutionalized mentally retarded citizens tend to be ill-equipped to understand or adjust to the complexities of life in the community. Whether based on the passive conformity fostered in large public institutions or the limited capacities of these individuals for managing more demanding sets of psychosocial expectancies, the response has too often been the same: bewilderment, poor adjustment, and, at times, major and prolonged emotional turmoil. This professional challenge has become acute as the number of public institutions for the mentally retarded has decreased dramatically during the last decade. Similarly, more attention needs to be focused on the various chronological age groupings of the mentally handicapped regarding their distinctive diagnostic and possible treatment spectrums. The recent sharp increase in societal awareness of the care given to elderly citizens—retarded or not—demonstrates our evolving professional interface with truly unique psychopharmacological challenges and treatment opportunities (Menolascino and Potter 1989a, 1989b).

CONCLUSION

Enhanced diagnostic understanding of the nature and types of mental illness in mentally retarded individuals has slowly begun to clarify those complex psychiatric disorders that we can or cannot effectively treat with the hope of obtaining optimum results. Such studies as those reported in this book on evolving psychopharmacology for mentally ill mentally retarded citizens illustrate a new interest in the single case-study approach, with its allied needs for increased research interaction, ongoing national pooling of results, and rapid dissemination of new treatment approaches (Agran et al. 1988).

Retarded citizens with allied mental illnesses still tend to fall into the gap that has traditionally separated mental-retardation services and research from those for mental health. In the past, the needs of dually diagnosed patients have gone almost totally unmet as both systems floundered in their interest or ability to address these challenges directly. Those who have been closely identified with the fields have striven for years to clarify the distinction between mental retardation and mental illness. They have been frustrated by the general public's confusion regarding the two conditions and concerned by the tendency of some health care professionals to apply mental-health approaches inappropriately to mental retardation. Fortunately, erroneous interpretations are increasingly viewed as largely representative of historical professional postures. The contributors to this book, by their attention to furthering our understanding of the treatability of the mental illnesses that mentally retarded citizens so often display, have helped to "close the door" on past restrictive psychopharmacological approaches. Their contributions stress the art of the possible in terms of how health care professionals can contribute to the developmental and general life enhancement of those mentally retarded citizens whose lives have been complicated by mental illness.

REFERENCES

Agran M, Moore S, Martin JE: Research in mental retardation: under-reporting of medication information. Res Dev Dis 9:351–357, 1988

Aman MG: Drugs in mental retardation: treatment or tragedy? Aust N Z J Dev Dis 10:215–226, 1985

Aman MG, Singh NN: A critical appraisal of recent drug research in mental retardation: the Coldwater studies. J Ment Defic Res 30:203–216, 1986

American Psychiatric Association: Diagnostic and Statistical Manual of Mental Disorders, 3rd Edition. Washington, DC, American Psychiatric Association, 1980

American Psychiatric Association: Diagnostic and Statistical Manual of Mental Disorders, 3rd Edition, Revised. Washington, DC, American Psychiatric Association, 1987

American Psychiatric Association: A Task Force Report of the American Psychiatric Association. Washington, DC, American Psychiatric Press, 1989

Beitenman ET: The psychiatric consultant in a residential facility for the mentally retarded, in Psychiatric Approaches to Mental Retardation. Edited by Menolascino F. New York, Basic Books, 1981, pp 527–541

Colodny D, Kurlander LF: Psychopharmacology as a treatment adjunct for the mentally retarded: problems and issues, in Psychiatric Approaches to Mental Retardation. Edited by Menolascino FJ. New York, Basic Books, 1970, pp 368–386

Day K: A hospital-based treatment programme for male mentally handicapped offenders. Br J Psychiatry 153:635–644, 1988

Donaldson JW: Specific psychopharmacological approaches and rationale for mentally retarded-mentally ill children, in Handbook of Mental Illness in the Mentally Retarded. Edited by Menolascino FJ, Stark J. New York, Plenum, 1984, pp 171–188

Fletcher RJ, Menolascino FJ: Mental Retardation and Mental Illness: Assessment, Treatment, and Service for the Dually Diagnosed. Lexington, MA, Lexington Books (in press)

Ghaziuddin M: Behavioral disorder in the mentally handicapped: the role of life events. Br J Psychiatry 152:683–686, 1988

Grossman H: Manual of Terminology and Classification in Mental Retardation. Washington, DC, American Association on Mental Deficiency, 1983

Jacobson HG: Positron emission tomography: a new approach to brain chemistry. JAMA 260:2704–2710, 1988

Lipton RS: The use of psychopharmacological agents in residential facilities for the retarded, in Psychiatric Approaches to Mental Retardation. Edited by Menolascino FJ. New York, Basic Books, 1970, pp 387–398

Lund J: Psychiatric aspects of Down's syndrome. Acta Psychiatr Scand 78:369–374, 1988

Matson JL: The PIMRA Test Manual. Orland Park, IL, International Diagnosis Systems, 1988

McGee JJ, Pearson PH: Personnel preparation to meet the mental health needs of the mentally retarded and their families: role of the university-affiliated programs, in Mental Illness and Mental Retardation: Bridging the Gap. Edited by Menolascino FJ, McCann BM. Baltimore, MD, University Park Press, 1983, pp 235–254

Menolascino FJ: Psychiatric Approaches to Mental Retardation. New York, Basic Books, 1970

Menolascino FJ, McCann BM: Mental Health and Mental Retardation: Bridging the Gap. Baltimore, MD, University Park Press, 1983

Menolascino FJ, Potter JF: Delivery of services in rural settings to the elderly mentally retarded-mentally ill. Int J Aging Human Dev 28:261–275, 1989a

Menolascino FJ, Potter JF: Mental illness in the elderly mentally retarded. J Appl Gerontol 8:192–202, 1989b

Montgomery G: The mind in motion. Discover, March 1989, pp 58–68

Reiss S, Levitan G, Szyszko J: Emotional disturbance and mental retardation: diagnostic overshadowing. Am J Ment Defic 86:567–574, 1982

Sonnander K: Early identification and prognosis: parental developmental assessment of 18-month old children. Ups J Med Sci Suppl 44:70–75, 1986

Sovner R: Limiting factors in the use of DSM-III criteria with mentally ill/mentally retarded persons. Psychopharmacol Bull 22:1055–1060, 1986

Sovner R: Behavioral psychopharmacology: a new psychiatric subspecialty, in Mental Retardation and Mental Health: Classification, Diagnosis, Treatment, Services. Edited by Stark J, Menolascino FJ, Albarelli MH, et al. New York, Springer-Verlag, 1988, pp 229–242

Stark J, Menolascino FJ: Training of psychiatrists in mental retardation. J Psychiatr Ed 10:235–246, 1986

Stark J, Menolascino FJ, McGee J: Ethical issues in the use of psychoactive medications in the mentally retarded, in Psychoactive Medications in Mental Retardation. Edited by Breuning R. New York, Plenum, 1984, pp 248–260

Stark J, Menolascino FJ, Albarelli MH, et al: Mental Retardation and Mental Health: Classification, Diagnosis, Treatment, Services. New York, Springer-Verlag, 1988

Watson JE, Aman MG, Singh NN: The psychopathology instrument for mentally retarded adults: psychometric characteristics, factor structure, and relationship to subject characteristics. Res Dev Dis 9:277–290, 1988

Chapter 3

TMS: A System for Prevention and Control

C. Thomas Gualtieri, M.D.

The epidemic of neuroleptic overuse among mentally retarded people is one of those tragic experiments that nature, or history, will sometimes play. For 30 years and as recently as only a few years ago, the simple fact of being mentally retarded and residing in an institution meant that one was treated, like as not, with neuroleptic drugs. The doses were high, the treatment went on for years, and there was little or no consideration given to the side effects that the drugs could have. Not too long ago, neuroleptics were the only psychoactive drugs prescribed to mentally retarded people.

Then things changed. Today, the prevailing attitude toward neuroleptic prescription for mentally retarded people is one of almost universal disapproval, and the frequency of neuroleptic prescription has declined precipitously (Hill et al. 1983; Lipman 1970; Sprague and Baxley 1978). We understand now that the difficult behaviors that once led to neuroleptic "treatment" were largely a consequence of intolerance and ignorance or the result of living conditions that were demeaning and oppressive. We appreciate that some mentally retarded people are victims of mental illness, but they are few, and if their problems must be treated with psychoactive drugs, there is almost always a better alternative to neuroleptics.

The move against neuroleptic prescription is only in part a consequence of unfavorable publicity, juridicial decisions, and the turning away from the "medical model." It is primarily a consequence of informed judgment about the severe side effects associated with long-term neuroleptic treatment, such as tardive dyskinesia (TD), tardive akathisia (TDAK), and the neuroleptic malignant syndrome. These serious problems were not well known 10 years ago. Now they add an inordinate cost to the medical monitoring of neuroleptic treatment.

The change is mostly attributable to the discovery that positive behavioral effects of neuroleptic treatment in retarded people, especially for a long term, have been vastly overstated. After years on neuroleptics, one usually discovers a patient who still has serious behavior problems and who progresses slowly, if at all, in his or her habilitative program; but he or she is also a patient who just cannot be weaned from neuroleptic drugs. Then, one is confronted with a double problem: not only is the patient's behavior still maladaptive; he or she is also addicted to these deleterious medications.

Finally, the change is attributable to the development of behavioral techniques, programmatic treatments, and new pharmacological agents that render long-term neuroleptic treatment obsolete. We have learned that most of the behavioral peculiarities that occur in mentally retarded people can be dealt with by teaching them better ways to behave or by adjusting their environment to be more understanding, more tolerant, or more accommodating. In the most difficult cases, there are psychotropics that work better than the neuroleptics (Gualtieri 1989).

It is as if drugs are like microbes that sweep through populations like an epidemic. The drug is a microbe, and the unwitting physician is the vector. There is a wave of treatment and then a wave of disease attendant on the treatment. Then the waves pass, leaving in their wake some broken lives. The neuroleptic era was, in looking back, an epidemic.

Like microbes during a plague, treatment epidemics do the most damage to vulnerable populations. In the 1950s and 1960s, when the neuroleptic era began, mentally retarded people were the most vulnerable population. There is no polite way to say it: They were treated like animals. The ideals of normalization, community living, and a respectable, gainful life seemed remote and outlandish. Mentally retarded people were oppressed and mistreated in so many dimensions that there was no resistance to the suggestion that they really needed major tranquilizers.

Today, we understand that new treatments may have unforeseen effects later, but the real significance of TD was not appreciated until 1979 (American Psychiatric Association Task Force 1979). The real significance of TDAK, a behavioral analog of TD, is only now coming to be understood (Barnes and Braude 1985). We have learned to be skeptical of the claims that are made now for new pharmacological treatments, such as the dubious proposition that clozapine is a neuroleptic that will not cause TD (Kane et al. 1988). But in the 1950s, when neuroleptics were first prescribed for mentally retarded patients, the fashionable phrase was "wonder drugs." What was noted was only the immediate benefit of the "major" tranquilizers, not their long-term price. That is history; it is understandable, but it was a tragic mistake.

Today, we know that a new technology cannot be engrafted on a professional community that is unprepared for its consequences. When neuroleptics were first introduced, psychiatry was a field devoted to interpersonal psychotherapy, and the idea of medical psychiatry was remote. On the other side, neurology was dominated by a sense of therapeutic nihilism. Thirty years ago, psychiatrists and neurologists were in no position to offer guidance to general physicians on the proper use of complicated compounds like the neuroleptic drugs. The prevailing standards of care were as unequal to the challenge of psychopharmacology as they had been to the challenge of psychosurgery 10 years before (Valenstein 1986).

We have since learned that psychopharmacology is a technology of unequaled importance in neuropsychiatry, but it requires special training and skill to exercise it well. We have also learned, painfully, that skill is not necessarily possessed by every man or woman who has a certificate from the Board of Psychiatry and Neurology. Psychopharmacology is really a subspecialty of psychiatry, just as epileptology is a subspecialty of neurology, and the proper use of psychoactive and anticonvulsant drugs for mentally retarded people requires subspecialty training.

The extraordinary potential of neuropharmacology has been tarnished by the weakness and clumsy behavior of physicians during the neuroleptic era and diminished accordingly, but it has not been extinguished. We know now that we need a generation of neuropsychiatrists who can manage this extraordinary technology. We must train psychiatrists who are doctors and who understand the brain map that underlies the serious neuropsychiatric conditions. We must find neurologists who appreciate that at least some behavioral conditions may have an origin in the brain. Most important, we must find physicians who can master the technology of drug treatment. Simply because there are still regions of darkness and ignorance, not all of neuropsychiatry is terra incognita. Intelligent, guided practice is possible, even for the most extreme disorders of behavior and emotional response.

Thus, the history of the neuroleptic era has been a paradox. As the field of mental retardation has been "demedicalized," and as it has turned away from the paternalistic, medical model of the old institutions, the use of neuropsychiatric drugs has actually increased to epidemic proportions. Now, even as we begin to appreciate the terrible consequences of the neuroleptic epidemic, we are actually turning to neuropsychiatry for guidance and for help.

POSTNEUROLEPTIC ERA

As we are fully within the postneuroleptic era, the things that we need to accomplish are clear. There are four priorities in the neuro-psychiatric approach to people with mental retardation:

1. To undo the consequences of neuroleptic excess, especially TD and TDAK.
2. To improve the treatment of epilepsy and the use of anticonvulsant drugs.
3. To develop special new treatments for serious neuropsychiatric conditions, such as self-injurious behavior, that afflict some people who are mentally retarded.
4. To guarantee high-quality care in neuropsychiatry for mentally retarded people in communities as well as in residential institutions.

The technology to achieve the first three goals is available today—not all of the technology, to be sure, but most of it. For the most part, we know what to do.

The state of knowledge with respect to the first three priorities has been described by Gualtieri (1990). In this chapter, I focus on the fourth priority—technology transfer to the clinical setting. In particular, I focus on the problem of neuroleptic treatment and the tardive disorders. In general, I focus on the quality of neuropsychiatric care.

CURRENT PROBLEM OF NEUROLEPTIC REDUCTION

Mental retardation has been well organized toward the reduction of neuroleptic prescription, and it has been, by the numbers, half successful. The field, though, has been victimized by its own success. As successive waves of mentally retarded people were withdrawn from neuroleptics, it seemed to become more difficult to withdraw new patients or even to lower their doses substantially. In many programs, we seem to have achieved a rock-bottom number, a substantial number of people who cannot simply be withdrawn from neuroleptics because they develop serious behavior problems when the dose is lowered.

By the same token, as more people were deinstitutionalized, it became more difficult to deinstitutionalize new clients. Increasingly, clients were returned to residential facilities by virtue of behavior problems in the community. Increasingly, residential institutions became clusters of people who were too unstable, behaviorally or medically, to succeed in the community. As monitoring psychophar-macology succeeded in getting many people away from medications that they really did not need, it also succeeded in identifying a core group of people with severe and refractory problems, who seemed to require institutionalization and maintenance neuroleptics.

Some clients who were withdrawn from neuroleptics during a long and arduous period would be retreated by community physicians, who were not sufficiently alert to the problems of neuroleptic treat-ment and who tended to respond to mild and transitory behavior problems with standing doses of neuroleptic drugs. Then, ironically, the clients would return to the parent institution, and the long and arduous process of neuroleptic withdrawal would have to begin again.

Finally, there has been a large influx of mentally retarded people, especially the mild and moderately retarded, into mental-retardation facilities from state mental hospitals. Here were people with serious behavior problems, and most of them had been receiving high doses of neuroleptics for long periods of time (Craig and Behar 1980).

What was recommended 10 years ago—gradual neuroleptic withdrawal for virtually all mentally retarded people who had been treated for a long term—no longer seemed relevant. The recommen-dation had been effective, and, as a result, neuroleptic prescription had declined by half (Hill et al. 1983). But the problem had changed, and one was compelled to develop new strategies for dealing with the new circumstances. The job was no longer something that could be mandated by administrative guidelines or juridicial decree. It was a more complex problem. It spoke to the needs of a group of mentally retarded people who could not seem to discontinue the use of neuroleptics.

It was not sufficient to say "Well, you see, they really need it." This was not, in my opinion, the problem of a group of people with specific, neuroleptic-sensitive neuropsychiatric disorders. This was, more like-ly, the problem of a group of people for whom continued neuroleptic treatment was a necessary evil, until some better alternative could be found. But it would require all of the resources of modern neuro-psychiatry to find those alternatives and all of the resources of modern technology to get those resources to the people who needed them the most.

This was also likely the manifestation of a syndrome referred to as a "behavioral analog" of TD in 1981 (Gualtieri and Guimond 1981), which is now referred to as tardive akathisia. It is a syndrome of motor restlessness, hyperactivity, and extreme dysphoria. There are four similarities between TDAK and TD: 1) TDAK may emerge, like TD, when a patient is receiving maintenance doses of neuroleptics.

2) TDAK is more likely to occur when the neuroleptic dose is lowered or after the drug is discontinued. 3) TDAK may be masked by higher doses of neuroleptics, but that is, of course, only a temporary solution. 4) Both TDAK and TD may, in some patients, ultimately "break through" (Barnes and Braude 1985).

DEVELOPMENT OF TMS

Some colleagues and I originally developed the tardive monitoring system (TMS) as part of a research program that was investigating the prevalence and course of severe TD in mentally retarded people. Its origins were in monitoring patients who were ultimately meant to enter research protocols. But the system had to be designed to monitor the quality of neuropsychiatric care as well. It was a self-serving decision that had an air of mutuality; there was really no way to do honest research in a facility until the basic neuropsychiatric requirements of patients and professional colleagues were first addressed.

But then the development of microcomputer technology for psychopharmacology monitoring and quality control became an end in itself. It was no longer just a way to advance the goals of a research project. What began as a research tool—to advance small, specific questions—grew into a method with much broader application. Our computer monitoring system for TD research began as a quick fix to facilities that might one day participate in research protocols. As such, it was a partial success. But as a method for addressing a much more entrenched problem, as a way to guide good neuropsychiatric practice, it has had better success.

The TMS is a fully portable microcomputer-based quality-control system that can identify problem areas in psychopharmacology and develop strategies for their solution. It is capable of monitoring the success of a consultation arrangement, thereby making consultants accountable for the outcome of their work. It is particularly good for developing skills in psychopharmacology in primary-care physicians, who are, after all, the ones who usually prescribe psychotropics and anticonvulsants in mental-retardation programs.

The TMS was first used in a small, university-based neuropsychiatry clinic that specialized in the care of patients with developmental disabilities and traumatic brain injuries. It has since been applied in three regional residential centers in three states and in one community-based program in a fourth state.

The system is based on a personal computer, and it uses conventional data-base software that will run on a 10-megabyte hard disk. It can, therefore, be mounted on a portable IBM AT computer and taken to a site, or it can be linked to the site by modem. Alternatively, floppy disks can be sent by mail or hard-copy printouts can be exchanged between the client facility and the project manager's office. The system can be integrated with many facility-based software systems, such as those that are used to keep up with client statistics or with pharmacy patient profiles.

The data base contains the medical records for all of the clients in a given facility. The record is in three parts:

1. Demographics—such patient information as age, race, sex, etiology of mental handicap, previous medical history, family history, and developmental testing
2. Clinical record—the salient findings from serial examinations, records of target behaviors, seizures, drug treatment, neurodiagnostic tests, dyskinesia examinations, and past and current treatment plans
3. Codes—used for classification, on the basis of demographics and the clinical record

The initial visits of the project manager to the client facility focus on consultations on immediate clinical problems, staff education, and development of the data base. If a fully integrated computer system is required, a programmer will usually have to spend some time making the systems compatible. The data base is corrected several times, the reliability of its data is appraised, and a system is developed for updating the data base for new patients, discharges, new clinical information, and future on-site consultations.

The requirements for long-term clinical consultation and staff education and for specific monitoring interventions are decided on the basis of this initial needs assessment. The code reports generated from the data base identify areas that require special attention. If, for example, dyskinesia examinations are inaccurate, drug-history information is unreliable, or seizure records or anticonvulsant blood-level records are not up-to-date, then remedial action will be necessary.

Code reports are generated at regular intervals, and they can demonstrate compliance or noncompliance with a recommended course of action. The project manager monitors this process. The manager also arranges consultation visits and staff education, as needed. He or she is available for telephone consultations in the interval between consultation visits. Hence, there is accountability on both sides.

The system has been developed on site, first in a neuropsychiatry clinic and then in regional residential centers in states that are remote from the project manager's home base. It has been designed for utility, efficiency, and ease and speed of operation.

The TMS is capable of generating research data, for example, concerning the frequency of such disorders as self-injurious behavior and TDAK. It can identify patients with specific syndromes, such as phenylketonuria or De Lange, for clinical trials or experimental treatments. It can also provide longitudinal follow-up information. New instruments for evaluation, such as the Self-Injurious Behavior Questionnaire and the Tardive Akathisia Rating Scale, can be developed on the data base; when they are established as sound and reliable instruments, they may be incorporated into clinical management.

It is better to light one candle than to curse the darkness. The TMS is a small candle, but it can illuminate the consequences of the neuroleptic epidemic, and it may even alleviate them to some degree. The lesson of TD is that technology like this is essential to manage and direct the technology of psychopharmacology. There are simply too many patients and too few competent neuropsychiatrists—too much darkness, not enough light.

APPLICATIONS OF TMS

What follows is a historical account of the development of the TMS in practice, with the results of three surveys for problem areas in psychopharmacology practice. As the system grew, it was expanded. Reviews for TDAK and suboptimal anticonvulsant prescription were added to the initial review for TD. The results are not presented as research data, since they were generated by a clinical quality-control system, not by a research system. The data, therefore, are only as good as the clinical information was to begin with.

Clinical Trials: Clinic A

The neuropsychiatry clinic (Clinic A) was established at a university hospital to provide psychopharmacology consultation to developmentally handicapped individuals who lived at home or in community-based facilities. The clinic was the main site for the first controlled TD-prevalence surveys conducted for children (Gualtieri et al. 1984) and mentally retarded people (Gualtieri et al. 1986).

The clinic was not a particularly good place to do TD research, though, for a couple of reasons. The thrust of treatment practice there was, naturally, in the direction of minimizing neuroleptic prescription. Therefore, every attempt was made to maintain patients on low doses of neuroleptics, if this class of drug was absolutely necessary. Even in this case, however, the physicians who worked there were dedicated to finding alternative drug treatments. Therefore, the number of patients at risk was low; although the clinic received 100 new patients a year for a 10-year period, the total number of patients at risk for TD by virtue of chronic neuroleptic treatment was only 76 (7.6%). The second problem was that patients who had TD were referred to the clinic by health care professionals who were aware of its special interest in neuroleptic-induced movement disorders. Therefore, although the number of patients at risk was low, the number of patients with TD to begin with was artificially inflated by referral bias.

In Table 3-1, I present the summary data from the TD survey that was completed in the clinic in October 1988. Of 76 patients at risk for TD, 29 continued on neuroleptic drugs. Twelve of the 29 had been established to have TD, by virtue of either movements apparent during extended neuroleptic "holidays" or "breakthrough" movements that were apparent even on maintenance doses of neuroleptics. There were 30 diagnosed TD cases, of 59 at risk and diagnosable—a TD prevalence rate of about 50%. Only 1 of the 30 diagnosed TD cases had severe and persistent TD, but one does not know how many of the patients receiving neuroleptics would be found to have severe TD if withdrawn from neuroleptics for an extended period.

The conclusions to draw from this survey are that neuroleptic use in the clinic is low (7.6%) and that most of the neuroleptic withdrawals have been successful. Tardive dyskinesia is common, but most diagnosed cases are mild to moderate in severity. Many of these cases remit over time.

The real usefulness of such a survey is not at one point in time but over time. The important comparisons will come when the survey is repeated annually. By then, more neuroleptic withdrawals will have

Table 3-1. Summary data from tardive dyskinesia survey: Clinic A

Category	Patients (*n*)
At risk	76
History of neuroleptic treatment	47 (62%)
Currently using neuroleptics	29 (38%)
Currently using neuroleptics: movement disorder	12 (16%)
Currently using neuroleptics: no movement disorder	17 (22%)
Severe and persistent tardive dyskinesia	1 (1.3%)
Mild-to-moderate tardive dyskinesia	17 (22%)
Movement disorder persistent	11 (14%)
Movement disorder in remission	6 (8%)

been attempted and more cases will have been accurately diagnosed. More people with persistent TD will have had an opportunity to remit. The true structure of the disorder will grow more apparent. Scientific information will accrue, and the course of clinical practice may be appraised in comparison to the baseline.

Having developed the method, however, we decided that it would be more fruitful to apply it in naturalistic settings. In a university clinic, issues of referral bias and special treatments may confound results. The next two surveys were conducted in large residential programs, where there had been a long history of neuroleptic prescription and modern alternatives to neuroleptics had been slow in coming.

Clinical Trials: Institution C

Institution C was a 360-bed state residential facility for mentally retarded people. It had received a recent infusion of persons from the state mental-health system, many patients who had been treated with high doses of neuroleptics for long periods of time. The need for a careful review of treatment practice and TD monitoring was clear to the administration, who contracted to adopt the TMS on a trial basis. The program was further elaborated, with monitoring for TDAK and for suboptimal prescription of anticonvulsants added to the original protocol.

In Table 3-2, I present the status of neuroleptic and anticonvulsant management as of May 1, 1989. This is a program with a major job

Table 3-2.   Status of neuroleptic and anticonvulsant management: Institution C

Category	Patients (n)
Total number	360
Never used neuroleptics	175
At risk	185 (51%)
History of neuroleptic treatment	67
Currently using neuroleptics	118
Currently using neuroleptics: movement disorder	39
Currently using neuroleptics: no movement disorder	75
Severe and persistent tardive dyskinesia	7
Mild-to-moderate tardive dyskinesia	19
Movement disorder persistent	18
Movement disorder in remission	1
Neuroleptic history: no tardive dyskinesia	43
No neuroleptic history: no tardive dyskinesia	175
Tardive akathisia	24
Review anticonvulsant pharmacotherapy	103

to do. Despite 2 years of attempts to lower neuroleptic doses and institute trial withdrawals, one-third of the residents were still on neuroleptics and half of the population was or had been at risk for neuroleptic side effects. There are two straightforward reasons for this problem: 1) the admission of new patients from the mental-health system, virtually all of whom had a neuroleptic problem, and 2) the readmission of old patients who had been placed in the community neuroleptic-free and were readmitted while using neuroleptics prescribed by local practitioners, usually for fairly minor problems.

There is another problem, though, which is theoretical—the frequency of what seems to be TDAK, a problem that emerges as neuroleptics are being withdrawn and one that makes it extremely difficult to withdraw patients from neuroleptic drugs. There were seven patients with severe, persistent, and debilitating TD, three of whom were still using neuroleptics. It is fair to assume that there will be many more severe and persistent cases of TD discovered when more of the 120 are withdrawn. Nineteen of the 67 patients who had been withdrawn from neuroleptics (28%) had TD, and 39 of the 118 patients who continued using neuroleptics (33%) had TD.

There were two new changes made in the monitoring program for work at this facility. One was a review for TDAK, and the other was a review for optimal anticonvulsant practice. The former is new and experimental, whereas the latter is straightforward.

The survey for TDAK is a novelty, since it has never been done in a population-based survey and there is no acceptable instrument for TDAK evaluation and monitoring. The two rating scales that we use for TDAK evaluation are entirely developmental and require revision on the basis of psychometric testing, so we were compelled to use clinical criteria, not rating scales. For the diagnosis of TDAK, we required the following criteria: 1) history of neuroleptic treatment, 1 year or more; 2) history or presence of neuroleptic-induced extrapyramidal disorders, acute exophthalmos-producing substance, withdrawal dyskinesia, or TD; 3) development of new symptoms of restlessness and dysphoria while receiving maintenance neuroleptic doses, when the dose is lowered, or after the drug is withdrawn (within 12 weeks); 4) persistence of the same for at least 6 months.

When these criteria were applied to the population of Institution C, 24 subjects were identified—5 of them with severe and persistent TD, 6 with mild to moderate TD, 7 using neuroleptics and with a history of TD, and 6 using neuroleptics but with no TD apparent. That is, 18% of the patients had withdrawn from neuroleptics and 9% of the patients were still on neuroleptics.

The second new review was for optimal anticonvulsant therapy. The category REVA/C (review anticonvulsant pharmacotherapy) was used to describe patients who met the following criteria: 1) more than one concomitant anticonvulsant; 2) anticonvulsant blood levels not taken or above or below the accepted therapeutic range; 3) prescription of archaic anticonvulsants, such as hydantoins, barbiturates, ethosuccumide, and bromides; 4) no documented seizure for at least 3 years.

The results of this review show 137 patients with active seizure disorders (currently receiving anticonvulsants) and 103 who are REVA/Cs. This appears to be a problem that will require almost as much work as the problem of neuroleptics. Of the 101 REVA/Cs, 16 are currently using neuroleptics. It is reasonable to suggest that at least some of these 16 will do well when they no longer use neuroleptics, after their anticonvulsant regimes are improved. This improved regime might consist of such psychotropic anticonvulsants as carbamazepine or valproate being substituted for anticonvulsants with behavior toxicity, such as phenytoin or phenobarbital.

Not all of the REVA/Cs require medication change. For example, after the REVA/C category was broken down and reviewed further, all patients receiving three or more concomitant anticonvulsants were reviewed by the attending neurologist and the neuropsychiatry consultant. Twelve patients were identified, and only in one case was polypharmacy thought to be inappropriate. In the others, there was a severe seizure disorder that could not be addressed by anticonvulsant monotherapy or the patient was in the midst of an anticonvulsant transition that was gradually seeking to establish monotherapy. There were, in all, 18 REVA/C-D patients, those who met REVA/C criteria but whose anticonvulsant status was clearly justified by clinical circumstances or who were in transition to monotherapy. That leaves 85 REVA/Cs with which to deal.

The advantage of computer monitoring is not that it tells physicians what to do. The advantage is that it can actually make unusual or extraordinary practice defensible, by implementing a regular and efficient system of peer review.

The further success of TMS will depend on its ability to monitor change in the structure of treatment over time, to establish priorities for clinical attention and pharmacological changes. Quarterly reports permit the evaluation of drug changes and policy implementation. There is built-in accountability, since review is so painless and the goals of review are so clear.

Clinical Trials: Community Program F

Community Program F provided an interesting challenge. It was a

91-bed residential facility that was "going community." Its campus was being dismantled, and the residents were being placed in group homes surrounding a program core. This metamorphosis is not uncommon, but this particular one was confounded by a fascinating twist. The facility had been on the grounds of a state psychiatric hospital. Although it was small, it had been selected to receive virtually all of the behavior-disturbed and psychiatrically impaired mentally retarded people from throughout the state. At one point, only a few years ago, the prevalence of neuroleptic prescription at this facility was 85%. A goal, then, was to deinstitutionalize a group of severely disturbed clients, most of whom had long neuroleptic histories. Another goal was to reduce the overreliance on neuroleptic drugs and to monitor clients for drug treatment and side effects. The baseline structure is presented in Table 3-3.

Five-sixths of the population at risk continue on neuroleptics. More than half of them already have signs of TD. Only 4 of 11 patients no longer using neuroleptics have signs of TD, but 1 of the 4 is severe and persistent and there are doubtless more of them buried among the people still using neuroleptics. Already, 9 patients with TDAK have been identified among the 66 at risk (14%). Among 36 patients with current seizure disorders, no fewer than 35 are REVA/Cs.

This kind of profile does not necessarily indicate lapses in the quality of care provided by the facility. Instead, it represents in large part a legacy from a much wider medical community, especially from mental-health care. This prototypical profile is a consequence of years of selective deinstitutionalization and neuroleptic withdrawal and attempts at anticonvulsant monotherapy. The drug profile looks worse

Table 3-3. Baseline structure: Community Program F

Category	Clients (n)
Total	91
Never used neuroleptics	25
At risk	66
History of neuroleptic treatment	11
Currently using neuroleptics	55
Currently using neuroleptics: movement disorder	30
Currently using neuroleptics: no movement disorder	23
Severe and persistent tardive dyskinesia	2
Mild-to-moderate tardive dyskinesia	3
Neuroleptic history: no tardive dyskinesia	6
Tardive akathisia	9
Review anticonvulsant pharmacotherapy	35

because the successful cases have been placed in their home communities away from the core program. Rather than speaking to the quality of care, the profile indicates the severity of the present problem and the expense that will be required to correct it.

UTILITY OF A PROFILE

The system generates reports like SMA-12s (sequential multichannel autoanalyzers), profiles that indicate areas of concern, areas that have been successful, and areas that will require closer attention. Like a laboratory screening instrument, this system is not definitive or diagnostic. It is a screen, a first look, a way to monitor, and a way to assess change.

The system is not only amenable to research; it requires it. The identification, on a preliminary basis, of TDAK as a problem afflicting substantial numbers of patients (12% at Institution C, 14% in Community Program F) demands the development of more reliable measures of the purported disorder and the undertaking of the essential validity studies. I believe that TDAK will prove to be a catastrophic legacy from the neuroleptic era, but the burden of proof is on us to prove that this is so.

In this chapter, of course, I describe surveys conducted as purely clinical exercises, with little heed to the conventions of controlled research—yet with special attention to the clinical requirements of consensus among colleagues and the rechecking of ambiguous findings. It is thus very interesting that we have come up with numbers that accurately reflect the results generated by more controlled research. For example, the overall prevalence of TD in the three programs is well within the range that is given in the mental-retardation literature: 39% at Clinic A, 33% at Institution C, and 53% in Community Program F. The prevalence of severe and persistent TD has rarely been addressed in the literature, so there are no grounds for external comparison. Nonetheless, there is an internal consistency: 1.3% at Clinic A, 4% at Institution C, and 3% in Community Program F.

The research, though, must be in the service of clinical care. If computerized monitoring is to be successful, it requires the cooperation of a large staff, and the staff members, in turn, must see concrete results from the system. The ideal system has computerized medical records and medicaid billing capacity built in, along with the capacity to monitor. It is essential to have clinical credibility first and then to develop research. In the second stage, research will serve the end of clinical credibility.

REFERENCES

American Psychiatric Association Task Force: Tardive dyskinesia. Washington, DC, American Psychiatric Association, 1979

Barnes TR, Braude WM: Akathisia variants and tardive dyskinesia. Arch Gen Psychiatry 42:874–878, 1985

Craig TJ, Behar R: Trends in the prescription of psychotropic drugs (1970–1977) in a state hospital. Compr Psychiatry 21:336–345, 1980

Gualtieri CT: Mental retardation, in Treatments of Psychiatric Disorders. Edited by American Psychiatric Association Task Force. Washington, DC, American Psychiatric Press, 1989, pp 3–178

Gualtieri CT: Neuropsychiatry and Behavioral Pharmacology. Berlin, Springer-Verlag, 1990

Gualtieri CT, Guimond M: Tardive dyskinesia and the behavioral consequences of chronic neuroleptic treatment. Dev Med Child Neur 23:255–259, 1981

Gualtieri CT, Quade D, Hicks RE, et al: Tardive dyskinesia and the clinical consequences of neuroleptic treatment in children and adults. Am J Psychiatry 141:21–23, 1984

Gualtieri CT, Schroeder SR, Hicks RE, et al: Tardive dyskinesia in young mentally retarded individuals. Arch Gen Psychiatry 43:335–340, 1986

Hill BK, Balow EA, Bruinincks RH: A National Study of Prescribed Drugs in Institutions and Community Residential Facilities for Mentally Retarded People. Minneapolis, University of Minnesota, 1983

Kane J, Honigfeld G, Singer J, et al: Clozaril collaborative study group: clozapine for the treatment-resistant schizophrenic. Arch Gen Psychiatry 45:789–796, 1988

Lipman RS: The use of psychopharmacological agents in residential facilities for the retarded, in Psychiatric Approaches to Mental Retardation. Edited by Menolascino F. New York, Basic Books, 1970, p 387

Sprague RL, Baxley GB: Drugs used in the management of behavior in mental retardation, in Mental Retardation and Developmental Disabilities. Edited by Wortis J. New York, Brunner/Mazel, 1978

Valenstein ES: Great and Desperate Cures: The Rise and Decline of Psychosurgery and Other Radical Treatments for Mental Illness. New York, Basic Books, 1986

Chapter 4

β-Blockers as Primary Treatment for Aggression and Self-injury in the Developmentally Disabled

John J. Ratey, M.D., and Karen J. Lindem

The challenge of improving the quality of life for aggressive and self-injurious developmentally disabled patients is twofold. First and of primary importance is the concentration on treatment strategies that alleviate maladaptive behaviors. Second, pharmacological interventions that impose negative side effects must be avoided, and nontoxic regimens, oriented toward rehabilitation, must be devised.

Rehabilitation emphasizes growth in areas of capacity that lead to maximum independence for developmentally disabled individuals; however, this level of treatment often is unattainable in aggressive patients. Aggressive behavior, or even a threat of an aggressive outburst, often prevents participation in activities. Day programming, social interactions, and even minimal demands to perform daily living skills are frequently not attempted if an outburst is expected. Treatment of aggressive patients then begins to center on protection of the patient and others, keeping the individual calm, and prevention of provocating events that serve as precursors to aggressivity. Limited exposure and participation in programming, social interactions, group activities, or individual instruction restricts an aggressive patient's daily experience. Aggressive behavior prevents exposure to normative activities, inhibits learning and growth, and thus constricts the quality of life of a patient.

A chronic state of overarousal, an inability to control impulsive actions, and cognitive impairments provide little for these patients to work with when frustrated or provoked. Often these patients are quick to react to environmental changes, adapt poorly to their surroundings or circumstances, and are intolerant of frustration, disappointment, or demands. Their inability to adapt to incoming stimuli suggests an already overloaded system (Miller 1960). An overloaded, overaroused

51

internal state adds to this hypersensitivity and hypervigilance and lowers the stimulus threshold further. This state is a setup for impulsive, aggressive behavior to occur and may be directed outward or at the self. Aggression or destructive behavior, as used here, encompasses acts directed toward others and objects, such as hitting, screaming, and biting, as well as self-injurious behaviors, including head banging, finger biting, and scratching.

Developmentally disabled patients are particularly prone to exhibit a chronic state of hyperarousal because of their cognitive impairments. Perceptual, memory, learning, and verbal deficits all add to the difficulty of such patients understanding their inner and outer world, thus leading to a hypervigilant, noisy state with a background of fear and uncertainty. Dearousing the chronic experience of internal noise increases tolerance to incoming stimuli and enables processing and integration of information. Dearousal may, therefore, increase tolerance and reduce aggressive outbursts and allow for gains in areas otherwise unapproachable. β-Blockers have been shown to be successful in the reduction of such overaroused states (Koella 1977). The habilitative effect of β-blocker therapy is seen in the progression of decreasing hyperarousal, decreasing aggressive outbursts, and increasing adaptation to daily activity. Decreasing aggressive behavior allows a patient to be more integrative with his or her environment, reduces concern over patient and staff safety, and shifts the focus of care from protective to habilitative. Gaind et al. (1975) demonstrated that behavioral therapy for specific phobias was more comfortable for patients who were treated with oxprenolol prior to behavioral techniques. Oxprenolol has been shown to improve symptoms of tension and well-being (McMillin 1973). The heightened state of arousal created by the specific stressor can inhibit learning during behavioral therapy or prevent a patient from attempting behavioral techniques (Marks 1976). Other anxiolytics, typically used to treat anxiety, also produce central nervous system (CNS) depression, which can negate the benefits of behavioral techniques (Gaind et al. 1975). β-Blockers, used as an adjunct to behavioral therapy, reduce the somatic elements of overarousal without depressing CNS activity or inhibiting learning. The β-blockers reduce negative symptomatology and promote habilitative behavior.

Treatment stratagems for reducing aggression vary greatly between behavioral and pharmacological approaches. The use of medications to treat behavioral problems in this population is often the option of last choice. A conservative approach to medication is, of course, appropriate; however, some aggressive and self-injurious patients are often unable to make gains without pharmacotherapy. Traditionally, neuroleptics or major tranquilizers are used to alleviate difficult or major behavioral problems. Emphasis has been on eliminating neuroleptics for aggressive behavior treatment and replacing them with safer, more tolerated, and more habilitative pharmacotherapy. β-Blockers are a conservative, nonsedating treatment for debilitating behavior in such individuals.

The preponderance of overarousal, impulsivity, ritualistic behavior, and aggression deny developmentally disabled persons their potential level of functioning and quality of life. In this chapter, we present the β-blockers as a promising nontoxic intervention. β-Blockers have been shown to decrease destructive behavior and enhance adaptive behaviors, such as communication and socialization. In this chapter, we outline the history of β-blocker use as an intervention for psychiatric disorders, including aggression and self-injury. Then we present our experience with β-blockers in mentally retarded and autistic patients, including preliminary results from experimental trials. Next, by emphasizing the orientation on rehabilitation in neuropsychiatry, we discuss how β-blocker administration is related to the new age of hypothesis formation and testing. Finally, we note the properties of β-blockers of interest to health care practitioners, including proposed mechanisms of action, half-life, dosage, selectivity, and metabolism. The efficacy of β-blockers for the treatment of aggression and self-injury is developed within the framework of consequent rehabilitative behavior.

DEVELOPMENT OF β-BLOCKERS IN PSYCHIATRY

The β-adrenergic blockers first became known to the medical community in the 1960s as a treatment for hypertension and angina pectoris (Goodman and Gilman 1986). Researchers found that β-blockers effectively reduced heart rate, cardiac output, blood pressure, and blood flow in patients with hypertension. In addition to controlling hypertension, some patients using β-blockers reported an increased tolerance to psychological stressors. Furthermore, some patients were found to react less intensely to stressful daily events, such as hectic schedules, heavy traffic, and deadlines at work. Patients reported becoming less upset, explosive, and anxious under circumstances that would have previously created emotional upheaval, agitation, or temper outbursts (Granville-Grossman and Turner 1966; Panizza and Lecasble 1985). This unexpected finding suggested to investigators that β-blocker intervention might reduce anxiety.

The relationship between phenomenological feelings of anxiety— such as shaky hands, pounding heart, sweating, dizziness, and breathlessness—and the physiological changes that occur in the body under stress—such as increased adrenaline production, vasoconstriction, and increased heart rate—has been known for some time. James (1890) wrote that anxiety is associated with sympathetic nervous discharge. Further, the experience of visceral stimulation has been suggested as the trigger for the sensation of emotion (Cannon 1927; Schachter 1964). Breggin (1964) further emphasized that visceral stimulation reinforces the experience of an emotion, such as anxiety. The somatic sensations of anxiety may thus be a consequence of sympathetic excitation.

The reduction of the physiological and phenomenological experiences of severe anxiety has primarily occurred through pharmacological intervention. Benzodiazepines have been the traditional pharmacological strategy for the treatment of anxiety and related symptoms. Granville-Grossman and Turner (1966) made the first structured comparison of the effect of β-blockade on anxiety. The results of their study indicated that propranolol at 80 mg/day for 1 week reduced autonomically mediated symptoms. Research soon became devoted to the relative efficacy of benzodiazepines and β-blockers for reducing symptoms of anxiety.

Early research comparing β-blockers and benzodiazepines demonstrated that β-blockers were effective for generalized anxiety disorders. Tyrer and Lader (1974) compared 12 anxious patients, 6 of whom were somatically anxious and 6 of whom complained primarily of psychological symptoms. Comparison of scores obtained on the Hamilton rating scale showed propranolol as effective as diazepam in treating somatic anxiety. Diazepam, on the other hand, was more effective than propranolol for treating psychic anxiety.

In addition to generalized anxiety states, β-blockers were introduced to treat anxiety when the somatic experience of anxiety interfered with performance. For example, β-blockers have been used to treat the acute reaction of performance anxiety affecting musicians (James et al. 1977; Neftel et al. 1982), public speakers (Taggart et al. 1973), and students undergoing examination (Brewer 1972; Conway 1971). In most studies, β-blockade reduced tremor and stage fright and improved performance. Most important, β-blockers did not appear to create sedation or interfere with performance.

The effectiveness of β-blockers in treating these common anxiety disorders suggested that β-blockers might be useful in treating individuals with more extreme behaviors. Granville-Grossman and Turner (1966) found that β-blockers effectively reduced anxious outbursts in patients with intermittent explosive disorder (IED). For these patients, stressors lead to the loss of control of aggressive impulses, resulting in assaultive and destructive behavior. Several open trials and case reports demonstrate the usefulness of β-blockers in the treatment of such dyscontrol (Atsmon and Blum 1970; Elliott 1977; Ratey et al. 1983; Yudofsky et al. 1981).

Atsmon began the use of β-blockers for agitation in 1970 when he reported on the efficacy of propranolol to help control the toxic symptoms of acute variegate porphyria (Atsmon and Blum 1970). Elliott (1977) led the way in his seminal report of seven patients with traumatic brain injury. In this open trial, he observed improvement in target symptoms of belligerence, explosive outbursts, and general irritability with administration of propranolol ranging in dose from 60 to 240 mg/day. Yudofsky et al. (1981) were effectively able to reduce rage and frequency of violent outbursts of four patients with generalized cortical damage.

Williams et al. (1982), in a retrospective case review of 30 patients with diagnoses including conduct disorder, IED, and pervasive developmental disorder, noted that 75% of patients improved when propranolol was given in daily doses ranging from 50 to 950 mg/day. Ratey et al. (1983) reported that propranolol reduced verbal and physical assaults, temper tantrums, and unprovoked rage outbursts in three patients—one mildly retarded, one moderately retarded, and one with CNS trauma. Greendyke et al. (1984) was able to decrease physical assaults in eight brain-injured patients with IED in an open trial setting with doses of propranolol of 520 mg/day.

Mattes reported two investigations of β-blockers for aggressivity. In an open trial comparison investigating predictors of differential response to propranolol and carbamazepine, improvements were seen in psychiatrist ratings of global improvement for both drugs in patients with uncontrolled rage outbursts without regard for possible CNS predictors (Mattes et al. 1984). Extending beyond propranolol, Mattes (1985) then reported on two cases of patients with IED whose violent behavior was reduced using another β-blocker, metoprolol. Frequency and severity of outbursts were reduced in one case, and the second case reported only one tantrum with amnesia within an 11-month period.

Jenkins and Maruta (1987) also reported a retrospective case review of eight patients who had been given propranolol in doses ranging from 80 to 300 mg/day. In these patients with IED, aggressive behavior decreased in six patients, and no change or slight worsening was noted in two patients. Of the eight patients Jenkins reported, three patients were mildly retarded and one was profoundly retarded. All patients had behavioral outbursts consisting of screaming and verbal threats with physical aggression directed at either patients or staff members. Dosages of propranolol ranged between 80 and 300 mg/day, and all received other psychiatric medications concurrently.

Three additional reports have investigated the efficacy of β-blockers to treat aggressive and self-injurious behavior in developmentally disabled persons (Greendyke and Kanter 1986; Greendyke et al. 1986; Ratey et al. 1986). In an open clinical trial with many participants, Ratey et al. (1986) reported on 19 consecutive patients, each with an IQ less than 50, who were treated with a mean dose of 120 mg/day of propranolol. Target behaviors of aggression, attention seeking, intrusiveness, and self-injurious behavior (such as head banging) were positively effected in 11 patients, 5 additional patients improved moderately, and 3 patients improved only slightly or not at all.

Successful treatment of negative behaviors is encouraging, as is the concurrent improvement of positive behaviors included in the reports of some investigators. Greendyke et al. (1986) reported improvement of assaultive behavior with the administration of propranolol in a double-blind, crossover, placebo-controlled study of 10 patients with severe dementia of organic origin. Propranolol was given at 520 mg/day for 11 weeks. Assaultive behavior decreased significantly, with 5 patients responding markedly and 2 responding moderately. Two patients had little or no change, and 1 patient was discontinued during the placebo phase. Positive behaviors, social interest, irritability, and psychomotor retardation were also assessed to compare behavior during placebo and propranolol trials, although no significant findings were obtained.

Further, expanding on the positive side effects of β-blocker treatment, Greendyke and Kanter (1986), in a double-blind, placebo-controlled study of pindolol for impulsive, explosive patients with brain disease or injury, reported a significant reduction in the number of assaults for patients treated with pindolol at doses ranging from 40 to 60 mg/day. Significant improvements in behavioral parameters of hostility, uncommunicativeness, uncooperativeness, and repetitive behavior were also seen for patients receiving pindolol; change in the level of lethargy was not found significant. The lack of intrusive side effects—such as fatigue, lethargy, and depressive symptoms—has been observed with β-blocker treatment in highly aggressive patients of all diagnoses and will be discussed further.

β-Blockers have also been shown effective for the severe behavioral problems of aggression and self-injury in adult autistic patients. In an open trial of eight adult autistic patients with severe behavioral problems of aggression and self-injury, all eight patients responded favorably to β-blocker treatment (Ratey et al. 1987). The reduction of target behaviors was dramatic, as all eight patients demonstrated large decrements or total amelioration of behaviors. Head banging was the most common example of self-injurious behavior, present in six of eight patients. All patients demonstrated major reduction, and two patients stopped their head banging completely. Neuroleptic use was also affected by the introduction of the β-blocker. Six of seven patients were able to have their concomitant neuroleptics tapered or eliminated, and one patient remained on the same dose (mesoridazine at 300 mg/day).

In addition to behavioral changes in aggression, positive changes in speech and socialization were noted with the onset of β-blocker treatment. Seven patients showed increased attention, decreased perseverative and nonsense speech, and more appropriate prosody. Of particular note was one patient who began to indicate needs verbally for the first time, one patient who remained mute but learned appropriate pointing behavior, and a third patient who learned to initiate an appropriate greeting. Of the eight patients, one patient showed no change in speech. Social changes occurred in all eight of the patients. Eye contact increased, as did capacity to interact with individuals and within groups. Patients began to communicate feelings, notice the absence of others, seek out staff, become less withdrawn and more receptive to behavior training, and develop a more friendly demeanor.

PRELIMINARY RESULTS: DOUBLE-BLIND, PLACEBO-CONTROLLED STUDIES WITH NADOLOL AND PINDOLOL

We have just completed two separate double-blind, placebo-controlled studies in California, New York, Maine, and Massachusetts, looking at the use of β-blockers to treat aggressive and self-injurious behavior in developmentally disabled patients. In both studies, participants were selected because their aggressive behavior had previously been refractory to other treatment methods. One study involved the use of pindolol, a lipophilic β-blocker. We investigated its effect on aggression and self-injury, as well as its habilitative effects, in 60 moderately to profoundly retarded adults between the ages of 18 and 55. The second study involved nadolol, a lipophobic β-blocker; 50 subjects participated. All subjects for this second study were aggressive, self-injurious adults between the ages of 18 and 55. All patients were screened for autistic behavior, and only those who met DSM-III-R (American Psychiatric Association 1987) criteria for autism were included for participation.

Before participation, all subjects were screened medically, with a physical examination, analysis of blood chemistry, and an electrocardiogram (ECG). Concomitant medications were held constant when patients began baseline measures and throughout the study. Frequency of aggressive behavior was screened, and only patients exhibiting four aggressive acts or self-injurious behaviors per month were entered into the study protocol. In the preliminary sites reported here, few of the participants received concomitant neuroleptics. In the study with pindolol, 1 of 14 subjects received a neuroleptic. Three subjects receiving nadolol and 4 subjects receiving a placebo in the second study concurrently received neuroleptics.

Five measures were systematically administered to assess efficacy. Our main focus was the reduction of aggression or self-injurious behaviors. By reducing the number and intensity of problem behaviors, we hoped to find an increase in more positive behaviors, especially those related to performance, speech, and socialization. Frequency and intensity of behaviors were tracked weekly with the Modified Overt Aggression Scale (MOAS) (Ratey et al., in press; Silver and Yudofsky 1987; Yudofsky et al. 1986). Overall ward behavior was measured weekly through the Nurse's Observation Scale Inpatient Evaluation (NOSIE), and general response to treatment was assessed monthly through ratings on the Clinical Global Impressions scale. To investigate performance, the Peabody Picture Vocabulary Test and the Vineland Adaptive Behavior Scale (interview edition) were administered at baseline and again at study completion.

Side effects were monitored continuously throughout each study. Blood pressure and pulse were taken before the administration of each dose; if either dropped below criteria of 90/55 millimeters of mercury (mmHg) or 55 beats per minute (bpm), the dosage was held and reattempted at the next scheduled dosing time. The dosage of study medication was reduced if blood pressure and pulse rates continually measured below the criteria. Side effects were minimal in both studies.

Pindolol for Aggression and Self-injury in the Mentally Retarded

In the pindolol study, subjects participated for 24 weeks, including 4 weeks of baseline measurements, 4 weeks of placebo lead-in, and 16 weeks of treatment, during which patients, medical staff members, and research staff members were all blind to medication. Patients were randomly assigned to receive either pindolol or a placebo. The dosage of medication was gradually tapered from 10 mg/day to a maximum dose of 40 mg/day.

Preliminary results of our first site with 14 patients are provided in Figures 4-1– 4-3. Figure 4-1 shows that in patients treated with pindolol, the average weekly frequency of aggressive and self-injurious acts measured by the MOAS decreased by 40.1% in the final month of the treatment phase compared with the placebo lead-in. Frequency of aggressive and self-injurious behavior decreased 12.1% for control subjects during this time.

Figure 4-2 illustrates the improvement seen in communication skills. The group receiving pindolol improved in this domain by 47.7%. Figure 4-3 shows that social skills saw the largest improvement, as the group receiving pindolol demonstrated an average of 61.5% improvement. Although control subjects also improved somewhat, they did not show improvements as consistent as those seen for the patients receiving pindolol.

Nadolol for Aggression and Self-injury in Autistic Adults

Subjects in the nadolol study also participated for 24 weeks. After a 1-month placebo lead-in period, patients were randomly assigned to receive a placebo or nadolol for the remaining 16 weeks of the study. Subjects initially received 40 mg/day of study medication and were titrated to 120 mg/day. Preliminary results of 14 subjects showed improvements in aggression, including assaultiveness, property destruction, and screaming. Figure 4-4 illustrates a 33% decrease in frequency of aggressive behavior in subjects receiving nadolol, whereas aggressive behavior in control subjects decreased by 6%.

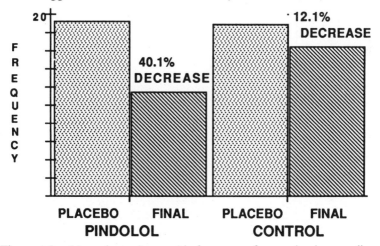

Figure 4-1. Mean change in monthly frequency of aggression in mentally retarded patients on Modified Overt Aggression Scale: pindolol versus placebo, preliminary results; $n = 14$.

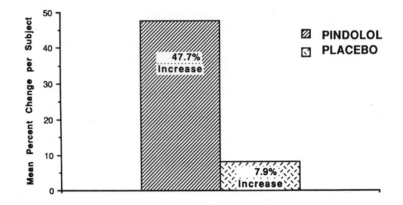

Figure 4-2. Improvement in communication skills of mentally retarded patients on Vineland Adaptive Behavior Scale: pindolol versus placebo, preliminary results; $n = 14$.

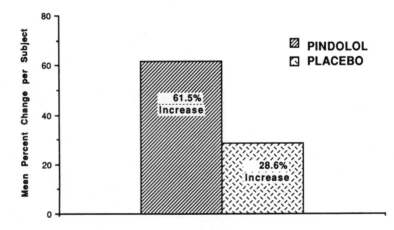

Figure 4-3. Improvement in social skills of mentally retarded patients on Vineland Adaptive Behavior Scale: pindolol versus placebo, preliminary results; $n = 14$.

Arousal and Performance

The main focus of these two controlled studies was the reduction of aggressive and self-injurious behaviors. By reducing the number and intensity of problem behaviors, we hoped to find an increase in positive behaviors, especially those related to performance. Gaind et al. (1975) reported that using β-blockers as an adjunct to behavioral therapy made patients less anxious and more comfortable. The dampening of arousal in overaroused states led to a greater chance for effective behavioral treatment. β-Blockers have been shown not to inhibit cognition or motivation (Betts et al. 1985; Harms 1985; McDevitt 1985; Panizza and Lecasble 1985). We also hypothesize that the action of β-blockers lowers the level of arousal in patients who are hyperaroused. Calming of this state, we suggest, will lead to improvements in learning, memory, and performance. Hebb (1966) detailed the critical features between arousal and cognitive processes. As illustrated in Figure 4-5, cognition relies on adequate attention to incoming stimuli. Low levels of arousal prevent the necessary attention to activate memory processes, leading to learning and performance. When activation is too high, attention to particular infor-

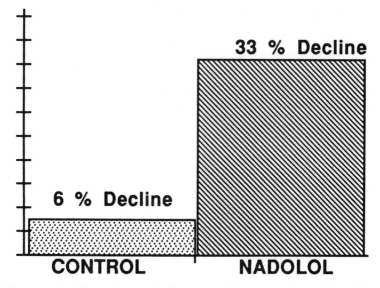

Figure 4-4. Mean decrease in frequency of aggression in autistic adults on Modified Overt Aggression Scale: nadolol versus placebo, preliminary results; $n = 14$.

mation is not attained, memory is impaired, learning is inhibited, and performance is constrained.

Patients exhibiting aggressive and self-injurious behaviors are functionally in a chronic overaroused state (Sands and Ratey 1986). As portrayed here, this state of overarousal inhibits the activation of memory, learning, and performance. The addition of a β-blocker, when arousal is at the upper end, will create a shift to the left, returning the state of arousal to a more effective level and optimizing cognitive functioning. This premise is the basis from which we promote the introduction of β-blockers for patients who cannot make progress in programs and activities because of overarousal, agitation, aggression, and self-injury. Central and peripheral actions have been supported in the literature as the mechanism for behavioral change. Benzodiazepines, neuroleptics, and other psychoactive drugs can also lower the arousal level. The central side effects of lipophilic β-blockers, however, are favored because they are mild compared with neuroleptics (Yorkston et al. 1981) and benzodiazepines (McMillin 1973; Tyrer and Lader 1974; Wheatley 1969).

Preliminary results from both studies support the hypothesis that β-blockers, as a less-toxic intervention, can reduce aggression and self-injury and promote the emergence of habilitative behavior. An important point and often-asked question is whether β-blockers are then only treating akathisia. Few subjects in both studies reported here received concomitant neuroleptics; therefore, positive effects resulting from neuroleptic potentiation or reduction of akathisia can be ruled out. In summary, a review of the β-blocker literature on open trials and controlled studies supports the use of β-blockers in treating aggression and self-injurious behavior for all diagnoses, including those in the developmentally disabled.

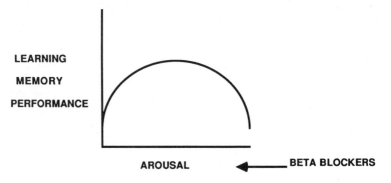

Figure 4-5. Hebb's (1966) learning and arousal curve.

MECHANISM OF ACTION:
CENTRAL VERSUS PERIPHERAL ACTION

Central and peripheral mechanisms have been proposed for the action of β-blockade for aggression and self-injury. Central mechanisms include specific blockade of the adrenergic receptors in the CNS, nonspecific effects on dopaminergic and serotonin systems, and CNS membrane stabilization. Peripheral mechanisms include interruption of β-adrenergic pathways, local anesthetic effects, and down-regulation of autonomic activity leading to lowered resting tension (Koella 1985; Sands and Ratey 1986).

Dopamine, norepinephrine, and serotonin have been implicated in aggression (Pradhan 1975; Reiss 1974). Agents that have an impact on and regulate these neurotransmitters are targets for possible antiaggressive drugs. Dopamine, norepinephrine, and serotonin are affected by blockade of the β-receptors. Serotonin receptor sites have been shown to be antagonized by propranolol (Weinstock and Weiss 1980; Weinstock et al. 1977). Reduction of central serotonin has been shown to reduce aggression in animal studies (Weinstock and Weiss 1980), although levels of β-blockade necessary to affect serotonin are obtained only at higher doses. Since central side effects have been reported to develop at high doses, it is unlikely that levels of serotonin are significantly affected by moderate doses of centrally acting β-blockers. Speculation about the key effect of β-blockade on each neurotransmitter is provoking but far too reductionistic, and it fails to encompass systemic complexities of the individual (Mandell 1986).

Stabilization of central membranes has been supported as a mechanism of β-blocker activity. Membrane stabilization, without acting on receptors, may regulate central activity in much the same way as anticonvulsants. The dextro isomer of propranolol has shown anticonvulsant effects (Leszkovsky and Tardos 1965). Dextro propranolol (d-propranolol) and conventional propranolol (dl-propranolol) have equivalent membrane stabilization activity (Atsmon and Blum 1978); however, in contrast to dl-propranolol, d-propranolol has only 1/60 the β-blocking action (Shanks 1976). The behavioral effects of the dextro isomer have been investigated in pilot and controlled studies of schizophrenic patients (Hirsch et al. 1981; Manchanda and Hirsch 1986). After admission, patients received haloperidol for 1 week. Those patients who then received d-propranolol were able to sustain behavioral improvements, whereas other patients did not. Neuroleptic potentiation was ruled out, because assays were therapeutically insufficient during propranolol administration.

The efficacy of d-propranolol noted in these studies implicates membrane stabilization as sufficient for behavioral change. Improvements in habituation and orientation have also been demonstrated with d-propranolol (Gruzelier et al. 1979); however, success in behavioral control has also been found with pindolol, which lacks membrane-stabilizing activity. Treating inpatients with organic brain disease, Greendyke and Kanter (1986) found significant improvement in aggressive behavior as well as communication and social behavior under controlled conditions.

A modulatory action in the limbic system has been further investigated as a possible central mechanism of β-adrenergic blockers. Propranolol has been shown to concentrate in the limbic areas (Massuoka and Hansson 1968), influencing the amygdala (Richardson 1974) and hippocampus (Garvey and Ram 1975; Ram et al. 1977). Neurophysiological evidence suggests that the limbic system monitors orientation and habituation responses to novel stimuli (Gloor 1960; Pribram and McGuinness 1975). Passive avoidance tasks require internal inhibition to withhold a response when a stimuli is presented. Response patterns on such tasks improved for patients receiving either d-propranolol or dl-propranolol compared with patients receiving phenothiazines (Gruzelier et al. 1978, 1979, 1980). The role of attention is considered by some to be a primary deficit of schizophrenia (Matthysee et al. 1979). Attention deficits are also an integral dysfunction for the developmentally disabled, particularly those who are aggressive. Pharmacological intervention that facilitates orientation and habituation beyond a sensory gating mechanism may also, as Gruzelier et al. (1980) pointed out, modulate other behavior and improve cognitive and social functioning.

β-Blockers may effect behavior via peripheral mechanisms. Changes in peripheral autonomic activity may account for some central actions of β-blockade. Peripheral feedback to the CNS has been shown to modify central activity. For example, an increase in sinoaortic pressure has demonstrated a reduction of central activity. In addition, indirect impact on central vigilance has been proposed by some, because extrabarrier structures are likely to communicate with infrabarrier structures (Koella 1977). Areas outside the blood-brain barrier may regulate central nervous activity through peripheral neural channels. Blockade of β-receptors in these extrabarrier loci, therefore, may have an impact on central autonomic systems through this indirect action.

Down-regulation of autonomic activity by the blockade of epinephrine in the periphery is an additional mechanism of action suggested for β-adrenergic blockers (Koella 1985). Neural and hormonal feedback channels, sensitized to decreased stimulation, transmit decreased autonomic activity to the CNS. Down-regulating the peripheral systems results in decreased arousal to the CNS (Koella 1985). An overtaxed CNS has been proposed and may be facilitated by dearousal (Polakoff et al. 1986; Sorgi et al. 1986). Regulation of arousal has been suggested to benefit particularly those patients prone to violent outbursts (Ratey et al. 1983; Sands and Ratey 1986).

β-Blockers also act on resting tension. Lowering the resting tension is an additional mechanism proposed for peripherally acting β-blockers (Lader and Tyrer 1972). β-Receptors are located on muscle spindles that set the resting tension of muscles. Blocking adrenergic activity at these sites thereby reduces muscle tension. This action on the resting tension of the peripheral musculature contributes to a state of lowered physiological tension, creating a general calming effect without inducing sedation.

Support of peripheral action is obtained from investigations of physiological tremor. Lipid- and water-soluble β-blockers have been shown effective in reducing essential tremor and tremor associated with Parkinson's disease (Foster et al. 1984; Herring 1964; Koller 1983). Many developmentally disabled individuals are secondarily tremulous, and this can add to aggressive and self-injurious behavior.

We have found that β-blockers cause many abnormal movements, such as physiological tremor, to be stilled with a concomitant positive effect on aggressive behavior. It has been proposed that motoric channels are a means of reducing an internal state of overarousal (Kinsbourne 1980). A state of internal hyperarousal, excessive stimulation, disorganization, and hypervigilance has been implicated in maladaptive behaviors, including stereotypies, self-stimulation, aggression, and self-injury (Kinsbourne 1980; Ratey et al. 1987; Sands and Ratey 1986). Internal "noise" (Sands and Ratey 1986) makes these patients prone to flooding, stimulus overload, and confusion.

Increased physiological stress, impulsive actions, and lowered ability to adapt to environmental change are consequences of an overloaded, overstimulated system. Goldstein (1948) demonstrated how ordinary stimuli provoke excessive reactions in brain-injured individuals compared with noninjured individuals. Brain injury, cognitive impairments, and poor impulse control add to the inability of many of the developmentally disabled to tolerate frustration caused by an inability to communicate needs adequately, function independently, or perform daily life routines. Behavior is then directed at reducing the state of overstimulation, with resultant dearousing behaviors, including stereotypical, aggressive, and self-injurious outbursts.

We suggest that the action of β-blockers for aggression and self-injury be viewed systemically. β-Blockers provide a chemical release from a chronic state of overarousal or noise that underlies many aggressive outbursts. Reduction of resting tension reduces the level of physiological tension and overarousal in agitated patients, thus creating a general calming effect. Blockade of peripheral norepinephrine feedback channels down-regulates autonomic input to the CNS. Thus, β-blockers provide the initial basis for a state of dearousal and prevent stress-induced autonomic reactions by reducing or regulating overarousal from sympathetic reactivity.

Thus, we can see the effects of β-blockers as bimodal in nature. First, following the tenants of the James-Lange hypothesis, we see that the β-blockers' effect on the body is crucial to dearousing a patient, as indicated by the sometimes immediate response of neuroleptic naive patients during the first week of treatment with nadolol, a lipophobic β-blocker. Nadolol, at the very least, requires attaining a high serum level and the passage of weeks before it accumulates in the CNS. Then the central action and its probable multiple actions on dopamine, norepinephrine, and serotonin systems occur secondarily. Thus, the cumulative effects of the β-blockers occur over a period of time. Gradual changes in behavior require a process of unlearning patterns of chronic behavior, at which time growth in adaptive behaviors, social interest, and appropriate communicative skills emerge. Treating the chronic state of hyperarousal seen in many mentally retarded adults with destructive behaviors is not proposed as a treatment of their primary deficits but as a treatment of the deficits that are possibly secondary to the central disease entity of developmental disabilities.

PRACTICAL GUIDE

Available β-Blockers

Currently, 10 β-blockers are available in the United States, each with different characteristics of liposolubility, metabolism, half-life, intrasympathomimetic activity (ISA), membrane stabilizing ability, and cardioselectivity. We have found that half-life, metabolism, membrane stabilization, and liposolubility are the most important properties to be considered in β-blocker selection. Table 4-1 provides pharmacokinetic characteristics to consider when prescribing β-blockers for aggression and self-injury in chronic populations.

Table 4-1. Pharmacological properties of β-blockers available in the United States

Compound	Trade name	Half-life (hours)	Elimination	Selectivity (β1, β2)	Partial agonist activity	Lipo-solubility	Daily dosing	Percentage of protein binding	Membrane stabilization
Acebutolol	Sectral	3–4	60% hepatic, 40% intestinal	β1, β2	+	Medium	2	26	+
Atenolol	Tenormin	6–9	Renal	β1	–	Low	2	3	–
Carteolol	Cartrol	5–6	50%–70% renal	β2	++	Low	1	23–30	–
Labetalol	Trandate	6–8	95% hepatic, 5% renal	β2	–	Medium	2	50	–
Metoprolol	Lopressor	3–7	Hepatic	β1	–	Medium	1–4	12	–
Nadolol	Corgard	20–24	Renal	β2	–	Low	1	30	–
Penbutolol	Ceratol	5	Hepatic and renal	β2	–	High	1	80–98	–
Pindolol	Visken	3–4	60% hepatic, 40% renal	β2	+++	Medium	2–3	57	+
Propranolol	Inderal	4–6	Hepatic	β2	–	High	2–4	93	++
Timolol	Blocadren	4–5	80% hepatic, 20% renal	β2	+/–	Medium	2–3	10	–

Note. Symbols refer to the strength of partial agonist activity: –, not present; +/–, weak activity; +, moderately strong activity; ++, very strong activity; +++, extremely strong activity.

Patient Selection

A patient who exhibits impulsive outbursts, who is likely to strike out unexpectedly, and who creates an alerted response in staff may respond well to β-blockers. A prototypical responder is difficult to define. A hyperactive, overdriven patient is the logical candidate, although often a retreated, emotionally withdrawn patient will also benefit from β-blocker treatment.

Symptoms that have been noted to improve with β-blockers suggest the type of patient who is likely to respond to this treatment. We have reported on two groupings of symptoms that improved when β-blockers were administered (J. Ratey et al., January 1987, unpublished observations). In our study with chronically hospitalized aggressive and self-injurious patients, we grouped symptoms of the brief psychiatric rating scale (BPRS) that had been reported in the literature as responding favorably. One symptom grouping included somatic concern, conceptual disorganization, emotional withdrawal, tension, and uncooperativeness. A second grouping of BPRS symptoms was specifically chosen to investigate effects on somatic tension and overarousal. This symptom group consisted of anxiety, emotional withdrawal, tension, hostility, uncooperativeness, and excitement. Other symptoms that improved included activation and hostility suspicion. Negative symptoms of schizophrenia, including uncooperativeness, social withdrawal, and blunted affect also improved. This suggests that patients who exhibit these behaviors may improve if treated with a β-blocker. Thus, patients who are overly active and overaroused, have low frustration tolerance, and are uncooperative and impulsive may be the best responders to treatment with β-blockers.

As with all drugs prescribed in this population, the most reasonable method to determine response is with an empirical trial. Setting objective guidelines to evaluate therapy response has traditionally occurred only under larger study designs. We suggest that this carry through to the individual patient. The dearousing effect of β-blockers may be reflected in the form of declined aggression along with improvements in adaptive behaviors. Setting up an empirical case trial requires the identification of maladaptive behaviors, baseline measurement of target behaviors, and longitudinal tracking from the baseline point through medication initiation and maintenance.

Exclusion Criteria

Medical History. Current medical condition and previous medical history, reviewed before administration of β-blocking agents, prevent most adverse effects from developing. Review patient histories for the following conditions, for which β-blockers are contraindicated (Williams et al. 1982; Yudofsky et al. 1981):

- History of allergy to β-adrenergic blocking agents
- History of chronic obstructive pulmonary disease
- History of bronchial asthma
- History of allergic or nonallergic bronchospasm—for example, emphysema
- History of congestive heart failure
- History of severe sinus bradycardia
- History of ventricular failure or cardiac shock
- History of insulin-treated diabetes mellitus
- History of hypoglycemia
- Current or recent (less than 2 weeks) administration of adrenergic augmenting psychotropic drugs—for example, monoamine oxidase inhibitors

Blood Chemistry. Liver and kidney functioning information and a general blood chemistry should be taken for medical screening. Total bilirubin greater than 2.0 mg/100 ml or serum glutamic-oxaloacetic transaminase or serum glutamic-pyruvic transaminase greater than 200 mg/100 ml; a history of hyperthyroidism or hypothyroidism as indicated by 3,5,3'-triiodothyronine, thyroxine, and total tritium; and a history of renal dysfunction defined as a serum creatinine greater than 2.0 mg/100 ml are indicative of abnormal liver or renal functioning. If these specific functions are abnormal, medications should be reviewed, and β-blockers should be initiated only after levels are within normal limits.

ECG and Cardiac Status. A current ECG should be reviewed to eliminate patients with a history of pathological cardiac conduction including arteriovenous block greater than first degree. The primary exclusions for the use of β-blockers are cardiogenic shock, sinus bradycardia with greater than first-degree block, and congestive heart failure. Our experience has shown that psychiatrists using β-blockers are conservative and tend to overexclude patients with borderline ECGs. This is not the case with the medical community at large, because some cardiac arrhythmias are treatable with β-blocking agents.

Liposolubility

Liposolubility refers to the ability of a substance to cross the blood-brain barrier and be absorbed by the CNS. If a compound is lipophilic, it will cross the blood-brain barrier easily and interact with receptors in the brain and CNS. In contrast, non-lipid-soluble or lipophobic compounds are unlikely to cross the blood-brain barrier. They are assumed to interact directly with the peripheral nervous system, although they may affect the CNS through feedback mechanisms and may be absorbed into the CNS over time.

Most psychiatrists, when talking about β-blockers, think and say "propranolol" or "Inderal" and expect that all other β-blockers are equivalent. Besides being the parent compound, propranolol is the most lipophilic β-blocker. Propranolol is active in the brain, blocking norepinephrine at receptor sites in the locus ceruleus (Koella 1977). Because of its high lipophilicity, it is quickly and thoroughly absorbed, a plus when the object is to maximize the amount of drug in the system and the brain. Several possible disadvantages also exist, however. Rapid accumulation of propranolol in the CNS may cause various side effects, including nightmares and other sleep disturbances and perhaps a higher incidence of depression and cognitive blunting, than do other β-blockers (Williams et al. 1982). In our experience, lipophobic β-blockers, such as nadolol and atenolol, have not been found to cause these central side effects.

Cardioselectivity

Cardioselectivity refers to the location of adrenergic receptor sites. β1-Adrenoreceptors are located primarily in cardiac muscle, whereas β2-adrenoreceptors are located primarily in bronchial and vascular musculature. All of the β-blockers have been found to act on β1-receptors. Most β-blockers have a greater nonselective action—they compete mainly for β-adrenergic receptors located in bronchial tissue and peripheral blood vessels. Atenolol, metoprolol, and acebutolol preferentially inhibit β1-receptors, although, at higher doses, they also inhibit β2-receptors (*Drug Facts and Comparisons* 1988).

Metabolism

Some β-blockers are metabolized through the liver, and others are excreted by the kidney unchanged. Thus, medications metabolized by the liver should be monitored when liver-metabolized β-blockers are used concomitantly. Important examples include neuroleptics and anticonvulsants.

Two studies have investigated the effects of liver-metabolized β-blockers on neuroleptics. Monitoring blood plasma levels of these medications is suggested. Thioridazine plasma levels increased three and five times in two patients treated concurrently with propranolol for destructive behaviors (Silver et al. 1986). Serum levels of thioridazine were shown to increase when pindolol was administered concomitantly. Serum phenytoin levels increased when pindolol was added to medication regimens of patients receiving phenytoin and phenobarbital concurrently. Serum phenytoin levels also increased if, in addition to phenytoin and phenobarbital, haloperidol or thioridazine was administered concurrently with pindolol. Serum blood levels of haloperidol, phenytoin, or phenobarbital did not increase if the medication was the only drug administered concurrently with pindolol. Serum pindolol levels were lower in patients receiving haloperidol, phenytoin, and phenobarbital than in patients receiving only thioridazine (Greendyke and Gulya 1988). β-Blockers, such as nadolol, pass through the body unchanged and are eliminated by the kidney (*Drug Facts and Comparisons* 1988). These β-blockers present the least concern when considering concomitant medications, because no competition is likely to occur.

Half-life

The length of time that medication maintains activity is an important characteristic for two related reasons—interdose rebound and dosing. Interdose rebound occurs because the half-life is short; missing a dose results in dysregulation, which is intolerable to these patients, who are overly sensitive to internal and external environmental changes. Dysregulation created by medication fluctuation is not tolerated, leading to a sensation of disequilibrium and imbalance, provoking destructive behavior.

The dangers of missing a dose because a patient refuses or forgets to take it plagues the shorter-living compounds. The experience of patients missing a dose and ending up with a greater degree of rage and self-abusive behavior led us to try the longer-acting compounds, such as nadolol and Sectral. A longer half-life is a benefit because it prevents interdose rebound from occurring and because dosing can then occur only once a day, decreasing demand on staff time during hectic dispensing periods.

Intrasympathomimetic Activity

Intrasympathomimetic activity is an agonist property that partially stimulates the β-receptor. The primary action of β-blockers with ISA is receptor antagonism, although the ISA property contributes by partially stimulating the receptor. Three β-blockers—pindolol, acebutolol, and timolol—have this additional agonist property.

Our experience with pindolol and acebutolol has demonstrated efficacy in treating aggression with these β-blockers. The combination of blockade and activation is crucial in certain individuals and could make these drugs the ideal choice. Because the property of ISA maintains some tone at the receptor, β-blockers with ISA are often effective for patients who develop hypotension while taking other β-blockers. In some patients, β-blockers with high ISA may act in much the same way as stimulants do for hyperactive patients; some individuals are calmed by this action, although others may be activated by the ISA. Therefore, behavioral improvement may be most significant at low to moderate doses when ISA is present. This partial agonist property is a delicate issue for psychiatric use. It is our experience that dosing needs to occur a bit slower and more cautiously with these β-blockers. Swings in behavior indicate that the ISA of the medication is too stimulating for the patient and the dose should be decreased or discontinued.

Dosing

Although the dose of β-blockers used is obviously important, we see the amount of time spent on a drug as a crucial variable and one that cannot be overemphasized. The dose used has to be tailored to the individual patient, because hypotensive side effects often limit the amount tolerated. Yet, even at low doses, positive effects on behavior can be noted, especially if viewed longitudinally. Psychopharmacologists are now attuned to the issue of time versus dose (Teicher and Baldessarini 1985). The "butterfly" effect (Lorenz 1979; Mandell 1986) of small doses for long periods of time may eventually lead to profound changes in behavior. Duration is perhaps most important for the seriously developmentally disabled populations. β-Blockers may initiate a decrease in noise and a quieting of the press for action. A decrease in aggression and self-injury may result quickly; however, a time lag may exist before behavioral patterns change. Old patterns of noxious behaviors need time to be unlearned and replaced with more habilitative behaviors.

Our experience suggests that behavioral changes can occur in the first month of treatment but may take as long as 6 months before the maximum effect can be noted. We propose the outline presented in Table 4-2, which is to be used as a general schedule when administering β-blockers.

In general, propranolol in doses between 40 and 360 mg/day are suggested. Many investigators have used doses much higher than this, although benefits from higher dosage levels are unclear because side effects are more prevalent. Although Elliott (1977) originally used doses at a maximum of 240 mg/day, most investigators have pushed the dose higher until the norm has been between 400 and 600 mg/day. The caregivers' press for rapid action in an aggressive and self-injurious patient is most responsible for the ratcheting up of the doses, which has led to the perception that higher doses are necessary to affect aggression and self-injurious behavior.

Propranolol should be started at 60 mg twice per day for 1 week and then titrated to 120 mg twice per day for 1 week and increased to 180 mg twice per day, ending with a total daily dose of 360 mg/day. Blood pressure should be taken daily to monitor for hypotension. Blood pressure less than 80/50 mmHg and a pulse less than 50 bpm have been reported as guideline criteria for hypotensive side effects (Williams et al. 1982).

We find nadolol to be two to three times more potent than propranolol, so its dosage should be correspondingly less, ranging from 40 to 160 mg/day. We have found doses of 120 mg/day most common; however, 80 mg/day may be effective if blood pressure drops below criteria levels. Doses of 40 mg/day have been noted to be effective.

Pindolol should be the easiest to use, because the ISA property supports the usual rate-limiting effects of blood pressure and pulse. Pindolol should be started at 5 mg twice per day for 1 week. As the dose is increased, in 10 mg/day increments, a paradoxical hyperactivity can occur. This requires slow increases and careful monitoring of the patient's behavior.

Withdrawal From β-Blockers

Patients who have responded well to a β-blocker, have stabilized their behaviors, and are being considered for withdrawal of medication should be withdrawn slowly. The nontoxicity of β-blockers enables gradual withdrawal. Reduction of total daily dose by one-fourth to one-third every month would be usual for these patients. In the advent of a side effect that requires immediate response—for example, bronchospasm, marked hypotension, or bradycardia—the β-blockers may be discontinued immediately, although heart rate and blood pressure should be monitored.

Peripheral effects are the immediate concern when discontinuing

Table 4-2. Titration schedule

| Compound | Milligrams per day | | | |
	Week 1	Week 2	Week 3	Maintenance
Propranolol	60	120	240	40–320
Nadolol	40	80	120	40–120
Pindolol	10	15	20	10–40

β-blockers abruptly. β-Blockers with the longest half-lives are the safest to discontinue immediately. The longer half-life enables gradual elimination, deterring rebound symptoms of tachycardia, hypertension, and behavioral dyscontrol. Nadolol is the safest to withdraw abruptly, because it has a long half-life and does not increase sensitivity at the receptor site.

Concerns about precipitation of a cardiac event with sudden withdrawal have been partially dispelled by recent evidence in the cardiac literature. Croft et al. (1986) investigated the abrupt withdrawal of β-blockers in patients with myocardial infarction. They concluded that abrupt β-blocker withdrawal did not increase the likelihood of rebound symptoms and, therefore, was not a major concern for these patients. Lindenfeld et al. (1980) also studied hypersensitivity to abrupt withdrawal of β-blockers in subjects without cardiac problems and patients with angina pectoris. Sympathetic hypersensitivity was not noted in either group of subjects after the withdrawal of propranolol given at 160 mg/day.

Summary

The difficulties in working with β-blockers are encouragingly few. Hypotension is the side effect most likely to occur, but it is monitored easily with each dose. A moderate decrement in dosage will normally alleviate unfavorable symptoms should they occur. The side-effect profile of propranolol is mild in relation to neuroleptics, although it can include hypotension, dizziness, nausea, sleep disturbances, and depression. In addition, lipophobic β-blockers have even fewer side effects to overshadow behavioral improvement. The work done with propranolol supports its use in psychiatric disorders, although evidence has been accumulating for the use of other β-blockers as well.

CONCLUSION

Although aggressive behavior does not interfere with all developmentally disabled individuals, intervention is necessary and critical for those who exhibit destructive behavior toward themselves or others. The complexities of behavior demand systemic strategies to create effective, long-lasting changes. Behavioral therapy and educational programs are often effective in modifying behavior; however, a substantial number of patients will never benefit from even these techniques, because the severity of their behaviors is peremptory to intervention.

Treatment of destructive behaviors must focus on the specific maladaptive behavior rather than the diagnosis or developmental disability. Aggression and self-injury are not diagnosis specific. The treatment of aggressive, destructive acts and self-injurious behavior is restricted if defined by diagnosis; it is not the developmental disability that is treated but the maladaptive behaviors of aggression. Head banging, finger biting, screaming, and physical attacks may have characteristics that parallel the outward appearance of psychotic episodes that formerly suggested the introduction of neuroleptics. Neuroleptics used as an initial or primary treatment choice is a limited option with questionable results and inevitable side effects. As neuropsychiatry broadens what we know of the brain and body's activities and reactivities, such a treatment choice will be considered only an accessory for aggressive developmentally disabled patients.

The treatment of aggression and self-injurious behaviors is difficult, because these behaviors are prevalent in vastly different diagnoses and treatments are frequently patient specific. The difficulty of treating aggression is further complicated because of the urgency of response necessary to keep patients and staff members safe. Such urgency promotes a potent medication; although it is necessary for an emergency situation, it is not indicated for chronic intervention. Treatment interventions must be interactive with an individual's daily life. Treatment of chronic behavior must be effective as well as tolerated over time. Pharmacological treatment strategies for aggressive behavior in the developmentally disabled must pay particular attention to cognitive blunting. Such medications as the neuroleptics can and do impair cognitive abilities. Impairment of cognitive functions further accentuates the disability and, in many cases, inhibits the use of existing capacities.

The β-blockers have continued to demonstrate their efficacy in clinical and controlled settings without inhibiting cognitive capacity. β-Blockers have demonstrated longevity, because they are well tolerated, produce few or transient side effects, and have noted efficacy. β-Blockers have demonstrated a calming effect for those patients who are intolerant of accommodation and whose impulsivity escalates in provoking or nonprovoking circumstances, leading to aggressive outbursts directed at others, objects, or themselves. We suggest that β-blockers be used for patients whose level of agitation and overarousal is intrusive to their daily lives.

Adult patients who may have exhibited many years of destructive behavior must unravel their set patterns of learned responses to the environment and overcome their inward drives for impulsive actions. The chronicity of overarousal seems to make the unlearning of these behavior patterns particularly difficult. β-Blockers decrease somatic hyperarousal as well as inner restlessness and tension that underlie the possible dearousing function of aggressive behavior. Once the hyperarousal is calmed, existing capacities can emerge, programming can be attempted, and progress can be monitored. Intervention with β-blockers is a more interactive pharmacological choice to treat aggression and self-injury.

REFERENCES

American Psychiatric Association: Diagnostic and Statistical Manual of Mental Disorders, 3rd Edition, Revised. Washington, DC, American Psychiatric Association, 1987

Atsmon A, Blum I: Treatment of acute porphyria variegata with propranolol. Lancet 1:196–197, 1970

Atsmon A, Blum I: Beta-adrenergic blocking drugs in psychiatry: present status, future approaches and research. L'Encephale 4:173–186, 1978

Betts T, Knight R, Crowe A, et al: Effect of β-blockers on psychomotor performance in normal volunteers. Eur J Clin Pharmacol 28 (suppl):39–49, 1985

Breggin PR: The psychophysiology of anxiety. J Nerv Ment Dis 13:558–568, 1964

Brewer C: Beneficial effect of beta-adrenergic blocking agents on exam nerves. Lancet 2:435, 1972

Cannon WB: The James-Lange theory of emotions: a critical examination and an alternative theory. Am J Psychol 39:106–124, 1927

Conway M: Final examinations. Practitioner 206:795–800, 1971

Croft C, Rude R, Gustafson N, et al: Abrupt withdrawal of β-blockade therapy in patients with myocardial infarction: effects on infarct size, left ventricular function, and hospital course. Circulation 73:1281–1290, 1986

Drug Facts and Comparisons. Philadelphia, PA, JB Lippincott, 1988

Elliott FA: Propranolol for the control of belligerent behavior following acute brain damage. Ann Neurol 1:489–491, 1977

Foster N, Newman R, Lewitt P, et al: Treatment of resting tremor by beta-adrenergic blockade. Am Heart J 108:1173–1177, 1984

Gaind R, Suri AK, Thompson J: Use of beta-blockers as an adjunct in behavioral techniques. Scottish Med J 20:284–286, 1975

Garvey HL, Ram N: Comparative antihypertensive effects and tissue distribution of beta adrenergic blocking drugs. J Pharmacol Exper Therap 194:220–233, 1975

Gloor P: Amygdala, in Handbook of Physiology, Section I: Neurophysiology, Vol 2. Edited by Field J. Washington, DC, American Physiological Society, 1960, pp 1395–1420

Goldstein K: After Effects of Brain Injuries in War. New York, Grune & Stratton, 1948

Goodman A, Gilman L: Pharmacologic Basis of Therapeutics. New York, Macmillan, 1986

Granville-Grossman K, Turner P: The effect of propranolol on anxiety. Lancet 1:788–790, 1966

Greendyke R, Gulya A: Effect of pindolol administration on serum levels of thioridazine, haloperidol, phenytoin, and phenobarbital. J Clin Psychiatry 49:105–107, 1988

Greendyke R, Kanter D: Therapeutic effects of pindolol on behavioral disturbances associated with organic brain disease: a double-blind study. J Clin Psychiatry 47:423–426, 1986

Greendyke R, Schuster D, Wooton J: Propranolol in the treatment of assaultive patients with organic brain disease. J Clin Psychopharmacol 4:282–285, 1984

Greendyke R, Kanter D, Schuster D, et al: Propranolol treatment of assaultive patients with organic brain disease: a double-blind crossover, placebo-controlled study. J Nerv Ment Dis 5:290–294, 1986

Gruzelier J, Connolly J, Eves F, et al: Effect of propranolol and phenothiazines on electrodermal orienting and habituation in schizophrenia. Psychol Med 11:93–108, 1978

Gruzelier J, Hirsch S, Weller M, et al: Influence of D or DL propranolol and chlorpromazine on habituation of phasic electrodermal responses in schizophrenia. Acta Psychiatr Scand 60:241–248, 1979

Gruzelier J, Thornton S, Staniforth D, et al: Active and passive avoidance learning in controls and schizophrenic patients on racemic propranolol and neuroleptics. Br J Psychiatry 137:131–137, 1980

Harms D: Visual reaction times may be improved by certain β-blockers. Eur J Clin Pharmacol 28 (suppl):51–54, 1985

Hebb DO: A Textbook of Psychology, 2nd Edition. Philadelphia, PA, WB Saunders, 1966

Herring A: Action of pronethalol on parkinsonian tremor. Lancet 2:892, 1964

Hirsch S, Manchanda R, Weller M: Dextro-propranolol in schizophrenia. Prog Neuro-psychopharmacol 4:633–637, 1981

James IM, Pearson RM, Griffith A, et al: Effect of oxprenolol on stage-fright in musicians. Lancet 2:952–954, 1977

James W: The Principles of Psychology. New York, Henry Holt, 1890

Jenkins S, Maruta T: Therapeutic use of propranolol for intermittent explosive disorder. Mayo Clin Proc 62:204–214, 1987

Kinsbourne M: Do repetitive movement patterns in children and animals serve a dearousing function? Dev Behav Pediatr 1:39–42, 1980

Koella W: Central aspects of beta-adrenergic blocking agents: mode and mechanisms of action, in A Therapeutic Approach to the Psyche via the Beta-adrenergic System. Edited by Kielholz P. New York, University Park Press, 1977, pp 11–31

Koella W: CNS-related (side-) effects of β-blockers with special reference to mechanisms of action. Eur J Clin Pharmacol 28 (suppl):55–63, 1985

Koller W: Nadolol in the treatment of essential tremor. Neurology 33:1076, 1983

Lader M, Tyrer P: Central and peripheral effects of propranolol and sotalol in normal human subjects. Br J Pharmacol 45:557–560, 1972

Leszkovsky G, Tardos L: Some effects of propranolol on the central nervous system. J Phar Pharmacol 17:518–519, 1965

Lindenfeld J, Crawford M, O'Rourke R, et al: Adrenergic responsiveness after abrupt propranolol withdrawal in normal subjects and in patients with angina pectoris. Circulation 62:704–711, 1980

Lorenz E: Predictability: does the flap of a butterfly's wings in Brazil set off a tornado in Texas? Paper presented at the annual meeting of the American Association for the Advancement of Science, Washington, DC, May 1979

Manchanda R, Hirsch S: Does propranolol have an antipsychotic effect? a placebo controlled study in acute schizophrenia. Br J Psychiatry 148:701–707, 1986

Mandell A: From molecular biological simplification to more realistic central nervous system dynamics: an opinion, in Psychiatry: Psychobiological Foundations of Clinical Psychiatry, Vol 4. Edited by Judd L, Grove P. New York, Basic Books, 1986, pp 361–366

Marks I: Psychopharmacology: the use of drugs combined with psychological treatment, in Evaluation of Psychological Therapies. Edited by Spitzer R, Klein DF. Baltimore, MD, Johns Hopkins University Press, 1976, pp 138–152

Massuoka D, Hansson E: Autoradiographic distribution studies of adrenergic blocking agents, II: C-propranolol, a beta-receptor-type blocker. Acta Pharmacologica et Toxicologica 25:447–455, 1968

Mattes J: Metoprolol for intermittent explosive disorder. Am J Psychiatry 142:1108–1109, 1985

Mattes J, Rosenberg J, Mayes D: Carbamazepine vs. propranolol in patients with uncontrolled rage outbursts. Psychopharmacol Bull 20:98–100, 1984

Matthysee S, Spring BJ, Sugarman J (eds): Attention and Information Processing in Schizophrenia. London, Pergamon, 1979

McDevitt D: β-blockers and psychometric performance: studies in normal volunteers. Eur J Clin Pharmacol 28 (suppl):35–38, 1985

McMillin WP: Oxprenolol in anxiety. Lancet 1:1193, 1973

Miller JG: Information input overload and psychopathology. Am J Psychiatry 116:695–704, 1959

Neftel K, Adler R, Kappeli L, et al: Stage fright in musicians: a model illustrating the effect of beta blockers. Psychosomatic Medicine 44:461–469, 1982

Panizza D, Lecasble M: Effect of atenolol on car drivers in a prolonged stress situation. Eur J Clin Pharmacol 28 (suppl):97–99, 1985

Polakoff S, Sorgi P, Ratey J: The treatment of impulsive and aggressive behaviors with nadolol. J Clin Psychopharmacol 6:125–126, 1986

Pradhan S: Aggression and central neurotransmitters. Int Rev Neurobiol 18:213–262, 1975

Pribram KH, McGuinness D: Arousal, activation and effort in the control of attention. Psychol Rev 82:116–147, 1975

Ram N, Hesse VC, Heilman RD: The effects of propranolol HCl in hippocampal lesioned rats. Arch Int Pharmacol 229:138–143, 1977

Ratey J, Morrill R, Oxenkrug G: Use of propranolol for provoked and unprovoked episodes of rage. Am J Psychiatry 140:1356–1357, 1983

Ratey J, Mikkelsen E, Smith B, et al: β-Blockers in the severely and profoundly mentally retarded. J Clin Psychopharmacol 6:103–107, 1986

Ratey J, Mikkelson E, Sorgi P, et al: Autism: the treatment of aggressive behaviors. J Clin Psychopharmacol 7:35–41, 1987

Ratey J, Sovner R, Parks A, et al: The use of buspirone in the treatment of aggression and anxiety in mentally retarded patients: a multiple baseline, placebo lead-in study. J Clin Psychiatry (in press)

Reiss D: Consideration of some problems encountered in relating specific neurotransmitters to specific behaviors or disease. J Psychiatr Res 11:145–148, 1974

Richardson JS: Basic concepts of psychopharmalogical research as applied to the psychopharmacological analysis of the amygdala. Acta Neurobiologica et Experimentia 34:543–562, 1974

Sands S, Ratey J: The concept of noise. Psychiatry 49:290–297, 1986

Schachter S: The interaction of cognitive and physiological determinants of emotional state, in Psychobiological Approaches to Social Behavior. Edited by Herman PH, Shapiro D. Stanford, CA, Stanford University Press, 1964, pp 45–66

Shanks RC: The properties of beta adrenoreceptor antagonists. Postgrad Med J 52 (suppl 4):14–20, 1976

Silver J, Yudofsky S: Documentation of aggression in the assessment of the violent patient. Psychiatric Annals 17:375–384, 1987

Silver J, Yudofsky S, Kogan M, et al: Elevation of thioridazine plasma levels by propranolol. Am J Psychiatry 143:1290–1292, 1986

Sorgi P, Ratey J, Polakoff S: Beta blockers for the treatment of chronically aggressive behaviors in patients with chronic schizophrenia. Am J Psychiatry 143:775–776, 1986

Taggart P, Carruthers M, Somerville W: Electrocardiogram, plasma catecholamines and lipids and their modification by oxprenolol when speaking before an audience. Lancet 2:341–346, 1973

Teicher M, Baldessarini R: Selection of neuroleptic dosage (letter). Arch Gen Psychiatry 42:636–637, 1985

Tyrer PJ, Lader MH: Response to propranolol and diazepam in somatic anxiety. Br Med J 2:14–16, 1974

Weinstock M, Weiss C: Antagonism by propranolol of isolation-induced aggression in mice: correlation with 5-hydroxytryptamine receptor blockade. Neuropharmacology 19:653–656, 1980

Weinstock M, Weiss C, Gitter S: Blockade of 5-hydroxytryptamine receptors in the central nervous system by beta-adrenoreceptor antagonists. Neuropharmacology 16:273–276, 1977

Wheatley D: Comparative effects of propranolol and chlordiazepoxide in anxiety states. Br J Psychiatry 115:1411–1412, 1969

Williams DT, Mehl R, Yudofsky S, et al: The effect of propranolol on uncontrolled rage outbursts in children and adolescents with organic brain dysfunction. J Am Acad Child Psychiatry 2:125–135, 1982

Yorkston N, Zaki A, Weller M, et al: DL-propranolol and chlorpromazine following admission for schizophrenia. Acta Psychiatr Scand 63:13–27, 1981

Yudofsky S, Williams D, Gorman J: Propranolol in the treatment of rage and violent behavior in patients with chronic brain syndrome. Am J Psychiatry 138:218–220, 1981

Yudofsky S, Silver J, Jackson W, et al: The overt aggression scale for the objective rating of verbal and physical aggression. Am J Psychiatry 143:35–39, 1986

Chapter 5

Use of Anticonvulsant Agents for Treatment of Neuropsychiatric Disorders in the Developmentally Disabled

Robert Sovner, M.D.

The efficacy of carbamazepine (CBZ), clonazepam (CLN), and valproate (VPA) in the treatment of neuropsychiatric disorders (McElroy and Pope 1988) has prompted their increasing use for developmentally disabled persons with behavioral and emotional disturbances. Treatment, however, is often directed at suppressing maladaptive behavior rather than addressing drug-responsive psychiatric disorders. This practice reflects, in part, the difficulties in conceptualizing mental disturbances in this population within a syndromic context. The DSM-III-R (American Psychiatric Association 1987) becomes increasingly difficult to use when the severity of an individual's developmental handicaps is moderate or greater (Sovner 1986).

The focus on the treatment of behavior also reflects the empirical tradition that has arisen in the use of psychotropic agents when working with the developmentally disabled. The management of aggression and self-injury has been of paramount concern, and a treatment model borrowed from behavioral psychology has been adopted (Sovner 1989a). In this chapter, on the other hand, I present a syndromic approach to the use of CBZ, CLN, and VPA. This approach may have great utility in predicting drug responsiveness in developmentally disabled persons.

RATIONALE FOR USE OF ANTICONVULSANTS

Anticonvulsants with psychotropic properties can, in many cases, be considered a treatment of first choice when all of the factors related to drug selection are taken into account.

CBZ, CLN, and VPA are effective in some cases of treatment-resis-

tant psychiatric disorders. Developmentally disabled persons, probably because of brain dysfunction (Roberts 1986), are susceptible to atypical and often treatment-resistant forms of classic psychiatric disorders, such as rapid cycling bipolar disorder (i.e., more than three episodes per year) (McElroy et al. 1988a, 1988b). Anticonvulsant therapy may be more effective than standard psychotropic agents in these cases (McElroy and Pope 1988).

Anticonvulsants with psychotropic properties can decrease the number of coprescribed drugs. Seizure disorders are highly prevalent in developmentally disabled populations—as much as 50% in individuals with severe or greater disabilities (Richardson et al. 1980). Consequently, the use of a drug with combined anticonvulsant and psychotropic properties can often eliminate the use of several drugs, thereby decreasing the risk of side effects and adverse drug interactions.

The side-effect profiles of CBZ, CLN, and VPA compare favorably with other psychotropic drug classes, particularly the antipsychotics. These anticonvulsants do not cause acute extrapyramidal side effects or tardive dyskinesia. The risk of severe adverse reactions (e.g., aplastic anemia with CBZ) is quite rare (Joffe et al. 1985). Also, these anticonvulsants (by definition) do not lower the seizure threshold, as do antipsychotics, heterocyclic antidepressants, and lithium ion (Itil and Soldatos 1980).

CBZ and VPA have relatively minimal effects on the habilitation process. Included in the risk-benefit ratio of any treatment for developmentally disabled persons is its impact on the patient's lifelong habilitation process. Drugs that impair learning and cognition can prevent the acquisition of new life skills and should be avoided.

CBZ and VPA have minimal anticholinergic effects (which can impair short-term memory) and minimal effects on cognition and performance (Aman et al. 1987; Gay 1984; Vining et al. 1987). CLN, on the other hand, is a benzodiazepine, and its sedative effects can be problematic.

MEDICOLEGAL ISSUES

Caregivers and advocates, who oversee the use of psychotropic drug therapy for developmentally disabled persons, often raise medicolegal issues when anticonvulsant therapy for behavioral problems is proposed. The recommended treatment is usually deemed to be "experimental," thereby necessitating a review by the facility's human research board. This concern generally reflects a misunderstanding of Food and Drug Administration (FDA) guidelines.

The FDA does not mandate the disorders for which a marketed drug can be prescribed (Archer 1984). The decision to use a specific drug, regardless of whether that indication is listed in the drug's package insert, should be made by the prescribing physician, the individual, and his or her advocates and caregivers based on the risk-benefit ratios of various types of interventions. Thus, it is not experimental to use an anticonvulsant to treat a psychiatric disorder.

A second and related issue is that the proposed treatment must be based on published research results. For the drug to be approved by the treatment team, the prescribing physician must provide studies documenting the agent's effects in the developmentally disabled. This is based on the assumption that the recommended treatment is specific for behavioral problems in disabled persons.

The clinician, however, should not have to demonstrate that the proposed anticonvulsant agent is an effective treatment for developmentally disabled persons any more than he or she has to demonstrate that penicillin is effective in this population. These drugs are not being prescribed as a treatment for the person's developmental disabilities but as a treatment for a superimposed neuropsychiatric disorder.

TREATMENT OF SPECIFIC PSYCHIATRIC DISORDERS

A basic psychotropic drug therapy principle in working with developmentally disabled persons is that psychotropic agents do not treat behavior per se but alter the neurophysiological processes that mediate it. In general, drug-responsive behavior reflects the presence of a neuropsychiatric syndrome. This means that the choice of drug therapy is determined by the diagnosis, not by the behavior of the developmentally disabled individual (see the section on mechanisms of action).

Clinical experience and research related to the use of anticonvulsants to treat affective disorders, panic disorder, and other psychiatric conditions are directly applicable to the symptomatic developmentally disabled patient. In addition, these agents may be helpful in treating psychopathology associated with organic brain disease even in the absence of a seizure disorder.

Treatment of Affective Disorders

Developmentally disabled persons suffer from the full range of affective disorders (Reid 1972; Sovner and Hurley 1983; Sovner and Pary, in press). Clinical experience suggests that this population may have a greater-than-expected incidence of atypical and treatment-resistant affective disorders, especially rapid-cycling bipolar disorders (Glue 1989; Naylor et al. 1974) and chronic mania (Reid et al. 1981; Sovner 1989b). This may be caused by increased incidence of central nervous system (CNS) dysfunction in general and seizure disorders in particular (Roberts 1986). Atypical presentations may represent subictal forms of epilepsy, which are particularly sensitive to anticonvulsant therapy (Blumer et al. 1988; Himmelhoch 1984).

Carbamazepine. CBZ has been the most-used anticonvulsant in the developmentally disabled for the treatment of affective disorders, and recent published experiences with the drug are summarized in Table 5-1. Signer et al. (1986) successfully treated a 34-year-old developmentally disabled woman suffering from a bipolar illness of type II (CBZ blood level was not reported). McCracken and Diamond (1988) treated five handicapped adolescents suffering from a bipolar disorder. Two had a rapid-cycling disorder, and one had a partial response to combined lithium, CBZ, and antipsychotic therapy. (One was also treated with thyroxine.)

Sovner (1988a) reported on the response of two patients with affective disorders. The first patient was a 25-year-old woman with autism, mild developmental disabilities, and major depression. When she had a major motor seizure with nortriptyline, the antidepressant was discontinued and CBZ was started. When her daily dose was titrated to achieve a blood level of 8.7 µg/ml, there was a dramatic decrease in anxiety and dysphoria and a remission in her sleep disturbance.

The second patient was a 21-year-old man with idiopathic mild developmental disabilities and chronic mania. (He had a positive family history for affective illness.) He had failed to respond to lithium or CBZ alone, but he had a significant decrease in manic symptom severity when the drugs were combined.

Glue (1989) carried out a point-prevalence study of affective disorders in 100 developmentally disabled adults who were in a long-term residential facility. He identified 12 residents with an affective disorder, and 10 of them had a rapid-cycling illness. Lithium therapy was initiated for 5 residents, but the drug alone was ineffective. CBZ was added in three cases. Two had a complete remission, and the third had a partial response (outcome measures were not specified, and therapeutic CBZ levels were not reported).

Reid et al. (1981) presented evidence that CBZ may be effective in organic mood syndromes in profoundly or severely disabled persons. They treated 12 institutionalized adults with severe or profound disabilities who manifested treatment-resistant and lifelong hyperactivity (5 had a history of epilepsy). The patients were treated in a double-blind, crossover trial in which CBZ and a placebo were each prescribed for 3 months. In the 6 subjects whose clinical presentation suggested chronic mania (presence of sleeplessness and euphoria), the mean weekly severity rating was significantly less for 5 of 6 study completers.

Clonazepam. To date, there have been no published reports of the use of CLN in the treatment of affective disorders in developmentally disabled persons.

Valproate. Sovner (1989b) presented five case reports of the treatment of bipolar disorders in persons with divalproex (an enteric coated form of VPA). Two patients had chronic mania, two patients had rapid-cycling bipolar disorder (one was also autistic), and the fifth patient had a classic bipolar disorder superimposed on an autistic disorder. These cases are summarized in Table 5-2.

Comments. There is sufficient clinical experience and research on the use of CBZ, CLN, and VPA in the treatment of affective disorders, in general, for anticonvulsant therapy to be considered a possible "first-line" intervention when working with developmentally disabled adults suffering from major depression or bipolar disorder. Considering the problems with lithium in the developmentally disabled—lack of response in some atypical cases, incontinence caused by polyuria, and the difficulties in managing weight gain (Schou 1989)—CBZ and VPA often have a better risk-benefit ratio for long-term therapy.

An issue to be resolved is the prevalence of organic mood disorders in developmentally disabled populations. Does the same brain dysfunction that produced the developmental disabilities also play a pathophysiological role in mediating these individuals' affective disorders? This may certainly be the case in rapid-cycling bipolar disorders, in which the presence of rapid cycling has been found to be independent of a genetic predisposition to bipolar disorders (Nurnberger et al. 1988) and to reflect brain dysfunction (Alarcon 1985).

The following recommendations are based on my clinical experience and the published reports on the use of these drugs as psychotropic agents; however, they must be considered preliminary until more data from controlled studies on the use of anticonvulsants in the treatment of affective disorders are available. Differential efficacy issues related to lithium, VPA, and antidepressant therapy are unresolved. The decision to use one drug instead of another must be based on illness and specific patient characteristics.

1. *Carbamazepine:*. CBZ has antidepressant as well as antimanic properties (Post et al. 1986). CBZ should be considered an antidepressant of first choice in unipolar depressed and disabled adults who have a preexisting CBZ-responsive disorder. I prefer CBZ for unipolar depressed autistic individuals, who may develop

Table 5-1. Published reports of carbamazepine treatment of affective disorders in developmentally disabled persons

Author	Patient	Psychiatric diagnoses	Clinical description	Response to carbamazepine
McCracken and Diamond (1988)	18-year-old man	Atypical bipolar disorder, moderate MR	1–2 weeks of hypomania alternating with 2–3 weeks of normal mood	He had attenuation of mood swings with carbamazepine (blood level between 8 and 12 μg/ml), lithium (2,100 mg/day), thioridazine (300 mg/day), and l-thyroxine (dosage not given).
Signer et al. (1986)	34-year-old man	Atypical bipolar disorder, mild MR	2–3 weeks of alternating periods of depression and hypomania; EEG was "nonspecifically abnormal" and CAT scan revealed mild cerebral atrophy.	Mood stabilization achieved (blood level not given)

Sovner (1988a)	21-year-old man	Chronic mania, mild MR	Patient had "several year" history of aggressive behavior, pressured speech, grandiose thinking, elated mood, and decreased need for sleep; he had not responded to lithium or carbamazepine alone; his mother had been diagnosed as manic-depressive.	There was a significant reduction in manic symptoms with lithium (.75 mEq/L) and carbamazepine (10.6 µg/ml).
	25-year-old woman	Major depression, autism, mild MR	Patient referred for an increase in self-injurious behavior of 18 months; she also had anxiety, mood swings, middle insomnia, and sadness; her brother had attempted suicide. Her pretreatment 4 P.M. DST was 16.9 µg/ml.	She had a major motor seizure on nortriptyline; on carbamazepine (8.7 µg/ml), depression remitted.

Note. MR, mental retardation. EEG, electroencephalogram. CAT, computerized axial tomography. DST, dexamethasone suppression test.

Table 5-2. Published reports of valproate treatment of neuropsychiatric disorders in developmentally disabled persons

Author	Patient	Psychiatric diagnoses	Clinical description	Response to treatment
Sovner (1989a)	24-year-old woman	BP-DIS, manic autistic disorder, early onset	Patient had a history of depression. She became manic during a decrease in daily thioridazine dose of 400 mg.	Complete remission was achieved. Thioridazine was discontinued. Maintenance DVP daily dose was 1,000 mg (VPA level, 78 mg/L).
	44-year-old woman with mild MR	Atypical BP-DIS, chronic mania, tardive dyskinesia	Patient had been manic for at least 5 years. She was taking thioridazine (500 mg daily).	Dramatic decrease in distractibility and pressured speech. Maladaptive behavior remitted. Thioridazine decreased to 100 mg/day. Maintenance DVP daily dose was 1,250 mg (VPA level, 70 mg/L).
	44-year-old man with moderate MR	Atypical BP-DIS, chronic mania, fragile X syndrome	Patient had been manic for at least 2 years. He was free of drugs.	Significant improvement in attention and concentration, with decrease in assaultiveness. Maintenance DVP daily dose was 1,000 mg (VPA level, 61 mg/L).

| 42-year-old man with mild MR | Atypical BP-DIS, rapid cycling, s/p alcoholism, tardive dyskinesia, s/p closed head injury | 6-day periods of mania followed by 2 days of normothymia and 2 days of depression. Mania would then return. Patient was taking haloperidol (5 mg daily) and lorazepam (2 mg daily). | Complete remission was achieved. Haloperidol decreased to 2 mg/day. Increase in severity of long-standing stuttering occurred during DVP treatment. Maintenance DVP daily dose was 1,500 mg (VPA level, 61 mg/L). |
| 31-year-old man with moderate MR | Atypical BP-DIS, rapid cycling, autistic disorder, early onset, s/p major motor seizure disorder | Manic periods lasting several days would occur every 14–21 days. | Normalization of sleep with remission of cycling; marked decrease in all target symptoms. Thioridazine reduced to 300 mg/day without relapse. Maintenance DVP daily dose was 2,000 mg (VPA level, 88 mg/L). |

Note. BP-DIS, bipolar disorder. s/p, status post. DVP, divalproex sodium. VPA, valproic acid. MR, mental retardation.

a seizure disorder in late adolescence or early adulthood.

With respect to bipolar disorder, CBZ is a reasonable alternative to or can be coprescribed with lithium (Post and Uhde 1986; Post et al. 1987). I have found lithium-induced diabetes insipidus and resulting incontinence to be a significant problem in persons with severe or profound disabilities who have an affective disorder and are being treated with this drug.

A blood level greater than 8.5 µg/ml may have to be achieved before a full clinical effect is observed, although some individuals will respond with lower blood levels.

2. *Clonazepam.* The use of CLN to treat the signs of acute mania represents a useful alternative to antipsychotics. Daily doses of as much as 16 mg have been used in nondisabled populations (Chouinard 1988).

3. *Valproate.* VPA may be a treatment of first choice for chronic mania and rapid-cycling bipolar disorder. The former disorder is not listed in the DSM-III-R, but Slater and Roth (1969) considered it to be a late-onset condition in patients with preexisting affective illnesses.

In my experience, a blood level between 125 mg/L and 150 mg/L may sometimes be necessary to achieve full therapeutic effects from VPA in cases of rapid-cycling illness or chronic mania. There is now anecdotal evidence suggesting that VPA may convert a rapid-cycling illness into chronic depression. This may necessitate concomitant antidepressant therapy.

Atypical Indications

An atypical indication in the present context refers to the use of a psychotropic agent to treat behavior and emotional complaints in the absence of a clearly defined (DSM-III-R) drug-responsive psychiatric disorder, such as major depression. The presenting complaint is usually severe and treatment-resistant maladaptive behavior, such as self-injury or aggression (Reid et al. 1978, 1984).

Maladaptive behavior per se can be a manifestation of alterations in mood and activity level associated with brain injury. Seizure-related mood and behavioral states (see the reviews by Gedye [1989a, 1989b] of self-injury and aggression associated with frontal lobe seizures), structural brain dysfunction, and neuroendocrine and metabolic disorders can produce pathological mood states (e.g., irritability), affective dysregulation (e.g., mood lability and rage), and behavioral disturbances (e.g., hyperactivity). Reid et al. (1984) aptly made this point:

nearly all severely and profoundly retarded patients will have major structural brain abnormality of some sort . . ., and symptoms such as abnormalities in levels of activity, distractability, lability, defects in emotional control manifested as irritability and noisiness, disturbed sleep patterns and persistent elevation of mood, are probably most appropriately regarded as brain damage phenomena. (p. 292)

These behaviors may be best considered as exaggerations or distortions of normal function rather than a state phenomenon. The behavioral presentation will depend on interaction among the site of the dysfunction, the age of onset, stability of the pathological process, and the individual's social learning history.

Carbamazepine. Reports before 1980 suggested that carbamazepine may have significant psychotropic effects. Donner and Frisk (1965) treated seven developmentally disabled children with severe epilepsy and an "organic psychosyndrome" or "neurotic symptoms" with CBZ. They reported that three of the children had a positive psychotropic response to treatment. Kanjilal (1977) treated 38 developmentally disabled epileptic patients with behavioral problems (restlessness, excitability, temper outbursts, aggression, or self-injury). His subjective impression was that 14 of his patients had improved behavior during the CBZ trial.

D'Hollander (1979) also found a significant psychotropic response to CBZ in 35 developmentally disabled and epileptic girls with behavioral disturbances. Dalby (1975), in reviewing earlier studies on the use of CBZ in disabled persons, cited evidence for its efficacy in the management of overactivity, impulsivity, and irritability.

More recent and detailed case reports have provided additional evidence to these effects. These cases are summarized in Table 5-3. Rapport et al. (1983) treated a 13-year-old girl with developmental disabilities secondary to measles encephalitis, a seizure disorder, and aggressive behavior. The combination of CBZ (blood level not provided) and behavior therapy produced a remission in her aggressive behavior.

Buck and Havey (1986) treated a 23-year-old man with mild developmental disabilities and a history of chronic and treatment-resistant behavior problems, including aggressive outbursts and talking incoherently to himself in the second person. He had nonspecific slowing on his electroencephalogram. There was a dramatic response to CBZ, with a blood level of 10 μg/ml.

Gupta et al. (1987) treated a 39-year-old woman with Prader-Willi syndrome, mild developmental disabilities, and a 25-year history of temper tantrums, aggressive behavior, and self-injurious behavior. Although they diagnosed their patient as having an intermittent

Table 5-3. Published reports of carbamazepine treatment of neuropsychiatric disorders in developmentally disabled persons

Author	Patient	Psychiatric diagnoses	Clinical description	Response to carbamazepine	Comments
Barrett et al. (1988)	11-year-old girl	Mild MR, r/o partial complex seizures	History of self-injury, foul language, and disruptive behavior.	Complete suppression of self-injury and growing, with blood level of 7.5 µg/ml.	Trial was double blind and placebo controlled, with crossover design. Behavior was probably not related to a seizure disorder.
Buck and Havey (1986)	23-year-old man	Mild MR	Chronic treatment-resistant aggression and incoherent speech	"Dramatic" response, with blood level of 10 µg/ml.	Patient's diagnosis was unclear.
Gupta et al. (1987)	39-year-old woman	Prader-Willi syndrome, moderate MR, intermittent explosive disorder	25-year history of aggressive outbursts; neurological examinations, including EEG and CAT, were within normal limits.	With blood level of 6.8 µg/L, there was a decrease in frequency and severity of outbursts.	Diagnosis of intermittent explosive disorder was not well established.

Study	Patient	Diagnosis	Presenting problem	Treatment/Outcome	Comments
Rapport et al. (1983)	13-year-old girl	Measles encephalitis, seizure disorder, unspecified MR	Aggressive behavior	Combination of carbamazepine (no blood level data provided) and behavior therapy produced remission of aggression.	Diagnosis was probably organic personality disorder.
Sovner (1988a)	27-year-old woman	Organic personality disorder, severe MR, congenital rubella syndrome	Patient had a lifelong history of irritability and hyposomnia associated with self-injury and negativism.	With blood level of 8.5 µg/ml, sleep disorder remitted and there was a significant reduction in maladaptive behavior.	Diagnosis of organic personality disorder was based on pervasive effects of patient's irritability.

Note. MR, mental retardation. r/o, rule out. EEG, electroencephalogram. CAT, computerized axial tomography.

explosive disorder, the data presented in the case report suggest that her aggressive behavior was caused by a low frustration tolerance and that an organic personality disorder would be a more appropriate diagnosis. She failed to respond to lithium or chlorpromazine but responded to CBZ with a blood level of 6.8 µg/ml.

Sovner (1988a, 1988b) treated a 27-year-old woman with severe mental retardation, bilateral cataracts, cardiac valvular defects, bilateral neural hearing deficits, and partial complex seizures secondary to a congenital rubella infection. She was referred for the evaluation of chronic behavioral problems, including self-injurious behavior, irritability, disrupted sleep, disrobing, and negativism. She had not responded to antipsychotic drug therapy. Her primary problem was believed to be a severe organic personality disorder with the primary features of irritability and hyposomnia. (Her self-injurious behavior and negativism were viewed as secondary features that served dearousal and demand-avoidance functions.) A remission in her sleep disturbance and a marked decrease in her irritability were achieved with CBZ (with a blood level of 8.5 µg/ml). Another benefit of treatment was that the four drugs that had been prescribed (chlorpromazine, haloperidol, phenobarbital, and phenytoin) were all tapered off without any loss of positive psychotropic effects or an increase in seizure frequency.

Barrett et al. (1988) presented a case report of the treatment of an 11-year-old girl with mild developmental disabilities, a suspected partial complex seizure disorder, self-injury, foul language, and disruptive behavior. She was treated in a double-blind, placebo-controlled crossover trial. There was a complete suppression of self-pinching and growling with CBZ alone (with a blood level of 7.5 µg/ml). Her neuropsychiatric diagnosis was not given.

Langee (1989) retrospectively analyzed the treatment response of 76 disabled adults who were treated with CBZ for treatment-resistant "behavioral disorders." Behavioral target symptoms rather than psychiatric diagnoses were used, and patients had to have significant behavioral pathology based on an index created by Langee (frequency of the behavior multiplied by its severity). CBZ blood levels were maintained at approximately 8.0 µg/ml. Thirty of 61 patients who met the inclusion criteria were rated as improved. There were no differences between responders and nonresponders with respect to demographic characteristics or the presence of a seizure disorder (27 of 30 compared with 23 of 31). Two CBZ responders who required additional lithium therapy were felt by Langee to be suffering from a rapid-cycling bipolar disorder. Reid et al. (1981), however, in the CBZ study of chronic mania (described in the previous section), found that overactive severely and profoundly disabled persons without signs of mania (e.g., euphoric mood) did not respond to this anticonvulsant.

Clonazepam. Freinhar (1985) reported a positive response to CLN (12 mg per day) in a mildly disabled 19-year-old woman with antipsychotic drug-resistant aggressive behavior and tantrums. No diagnosis was given.

Valproate. There have been no reports of the use of valproate for the treatment of atypical disorders in developmentally disabled persons.

Comments. The behavioral disturbances seen in developmentally disabled adults can also be seen in other brain-injured populations, suggesting that it is the brain injury, not the age of onset, that is the most important factor. These behavioral disturbances include irritability, mood lability, impulsivity, sleep disturbances, and aggression (McAllister 1985; McAllister and Price 1987; McQuiston et al. 1987). In some cases, they have proven responsive to CBZ (Devinsky and Bear 1984; Marin and Greenwald 1989; Patterson 1987). The presence of disrupted sleep (in the absence of an affective disorder) may be a good predictor of CBZ responsiveness.

It is interesting that Papez (1937) partly based his hypothesis that the limbic system mediated emotion on observations that the prodromal behavior of humans infected with the rabies virus included irritability, insomnia, and restlessness. These behaviors are often seen in profoundly and severely disabled individuals (Reid et al. 1978). Such findings suggest that the search for specific behavioral syndromes possibly associated with specific types of causes of developmental disabilities (e.g., viral encephalitis) may be a fruitful area for future research.

With affective disorders, a clinician simply has to see past developmental disabilities and their influence on symptom presentation (Sovner 1986). In the case of atypical indications, however, there is no diagnostic frame of reference. Treatment at this time is largely empirical but should be based on a set of target behaviors that are considered drug-responsive by virtue of their relationship to a patient's organic brain disease (e.g., rage attacks).

MECHANISMS OF ACTION

Maladaptive behavior serves various functions, including environmental control (e.g., demand-avoidance behavior), modulation of sensory input (e.g., self-stimulatory behavior in autistic individuals [Ratey et al. 1987]), and the amelioration of anxiety (Ratey et al. 1989). It is, therefore, simplistic to posit a specific drug response for complex behaviors—such as aggression, self-injury, and tantrums—

because they are final common pathways expressing not only neurobiological dysfunction but also psychological distress and attempts to control one's social milieu.

It is more relevant to look for a more primary psychobiological factor mediating maladaptive behavior, which can also serve as a bridge between pathophysiology and complex behavior. For example, a profoundly disabled hyperactive individual may become agitated when prevented from roaming at will and engage in aggression or self-injury. In addition, an individual with severe attentional problems, who relies on health care providers to provide direction and structure, may engage in attention-getting aggression when a favorite staff member is unavailable to provide supervision because of other pressing demands.

With these issues in mind, there are several possible mechanisms that may mediate the therapeutic behavioral effects of anticonvulsant therapy, especially in atypical cases.

1. *An undiagnosed "classic" psychiatric disorder is responsible for the patient's maladaptive behavior and is anticonvulsant-responsive.* Self-injury and aggression can be the presenting complaint in an affective disorder (Sovner and Pary, in press), for example. Based on preliminary work with buspirone (Ratey et al. 1989), the antianxiety effects of CLN (Greenblatt et al. 1987) should be considered as a possible mechanism of action in some cases of maladaptive behavior. It also seems likely that panic attacks could be responsible for paroxysmal self-injury or aggression. Thus, the administration of an anticonvulsant with psychotropic properties might remove the source of an individual's psychological distress.

2. *An unrecognized seizure disorder is responsible for the patient's maladaptive behavior and is stabilized with anticonvulsant therapy.* Gedye (1989a, 1989b) reviewed the literature on the behavioral manifestations of frontal lobe seizures and presented case-report data on seizure-related self-injury and aggression (the behavior is usually paroxysmal and associated with ocular manifestations, such as roll up of the eyes). Also, preictal or postictal irritability might result in aggression or self-injury. Thus, the stabilization of an individual's seizure disorder may produce a positive behavioral effect (Blumer et al. 1988).

3. *CBZ, CLN, and VPA specifically alter those neurotransmitter systems mediating primary organic psychopathology.* Hyperactivity, attentional deficits, irritability, impulsivity, and rage attacks can be primary behavioral manifestations of CNS pathology and may be mediated by specific dysfunctions in neurotransmitter systems. To

date, clear-cut relationships between various pharmacological effects of CBZ, CLN, and VPA and specific psychobiological dysfunctions have not been demonstrated, partly because of the diversity of effects of these drugs.

CBZ affects γ-aminobutyric acid (GABA), indolaminergic function, and catecholaminergic function (Post 1988). CLN has specific effects similar to those of other benzodiazepines and may also affect serotonergic function (Greenblatt et al. 1987). VPA primarily alters "GABAergic" function (McElroy et al. 1988b). Consequently, it is difficult to point to one pharmacological effect as the therapeutic one. However, the use of such drugs as trazodone to control agitation in demented persons (Simpson and Foster 1986) and tricyclic antidepressants to control mood lability in persons with brain dysfunction (Ross and Stewart 1987) suggests serotonergic and noradrenergic mechanisms are involved in mediating some anticonvulsants' therapeutic effects.

ADVERSE EFFECTS

Carbamazepine

CBZ is well tolerated by developmentally disabled persons (Bird et al. 1966), and agranulocytosis is a rare adverse reaction (Joffe et al. 1985); however, behavioral side effects can develop. Silverstein et al. (1982) found that 7 of 200 children treated with CBZ (3.5%) had adverse behavioral reactions to the drug. Four of the children were developmentally disabled (ranging in age from 6 to 18 years). Drug-induced agitation or irritability appeared to be the common denominator in these cases.

CBZ toxic blood levels have also been implicated in producing a schizophreniform psychosis (Franks and Richter 1979) and reversible dystonia in disabled children with epilepsy (Crosley and Swender 1979). The combination of lithium and CBZ can produce a neurotoxic syndrome, even when the blood levels of both drugs are within the therapeutic range (Shukla et al. 1984). Central nervous system dysfunction appears to be a mediating factor in all of these idiosyncratic reactions (Rivinus 1982; Shukla et al. 1984).

In a retrospective study of CBZ for the treatment of "behavioral disorders" (Langee 1989), the frequency of adverse reactions in 76 institutionalized individuals was as follows: one case with a leukocyte count less than 2,500 during the first 2 weeks of treatment; one case of severe dermatitis; one case of hyponatremia and "bone marrow depression"; one case of nausea (associated with elevated liver enzymes); two cases of ataxia (associated with an elevated phenytoin level).

CBZ induction of mania or an amphetamine reaction should be considered in individuals whose behavior deteriorates after therapy is initiated (Myers and Carrera 1989; Pleak et al. 1988). This is not surprising given the structural similarities between CBZ and the tricyclic antidepressant imipramine. Tricyclics have been associated with the precipitation of mania (Wehr and Goodwin 1987) and amphetaminelike reactions (Pollack and Rosenbaum 1987).

The effect of CBZ in increasing the metabolism of VPA is a clinically significant drug interaction, especially when attempting to substitute VPA for CBZ. In one case, I had to prescribe 6,000 mg per day of VPA to achieve a blood level of 50 mg/L while the patient was taking CBZ (Sovner 1988c).

Clonazepam

CLN is a long-acting benzodiazepine; it can be sedating and disinhibiting (Chouinard 1988). These adverse effects may limit its use in the developmentally disabled.

Valproate

In my experience, acute VPA nausea and diarrhea, long-term weight gain, and the potentiation of antipsychotic-induced tremor are the most difficult side effects to manage. Severe liver dysfunction and blood dyscrasias are rare side effects with valproic acid (Browne 1980). VPA has been reported to cause nocturnal enuresis in children (Choonara 1985; Panayiotopoulos 1985) and hyperammonemia in mentally retarded adults (Williams et al. 1984); however, VPA seems to have few adverse effects on learning in this population (Gay 1984).

CONCLUSION

CBZ, CLN, and VPA are valuable agents in the treatment of neuropsychiatric disorders in developmentally disabled persons. Clinicians must, however, consider the possibility that a patient's maladaptive behavior (or its increase in severity) is secondary to major depression and bipolar disorder of a nonaffective organic brain syndrome.

The use of anticonvulsant therapy to treat affective disorders is not particularly controversial. Its use, however, in the treatment of maladaptive behavior is much more problematic; there are no methodologically sound studies from which to draw definitive conclusions or models to be borrowed from general psychiatry. (The treatment of behavior problems related to CNS dysfunction in the developmentally disabled may turn out to be a model for the management of such problems in nondisabled brain-damaged persons.)

This does not mean that the psychotropic effects of CBZ, CLN, and VPA should not be used for atypical indications. The case-study literature is highly suggestive and argues for their use on a case-by-case basis, especially in severely and profoundly disabled individuals who manifest significant maladaptive behavior, which may reflect an underlying affective disorder or organic brain syndrome. There is reason to hope that the increasing experience with these drugs will produce clear-cut behavioral patterns that will guide treatment recommendations.

REFERENCES

Alarcon RD: Rapid cycling affective disorders: a clinical review. Compr Psychiatry 26:522–540, 1985

Aman MG, Werry JS, Paxton JW, et al: Effect of sodium valproate on psychomotor performance in children as a function of dose, fluctuations in concentration, and diagnosis. Epilepsia 28:115–124, 1987

American Psychiatric Association: Diagnostic and Statistical Manual of Mental Disorders, 3rd Edition, Revised. Washington, DC, American Psychiatric Association, 1987

Archer JD: The FDA does not approve the uses of drugs (editorial). JAMA 252:1054–1055, 1984

Barrett RP, Payton JB, Burkhart JE: Treatment of self-injury and disruptive behavior with carbamazepine (Tegretol) and behavior therapy. J Multihandicap Person 1:79–92, 1988

Bird CAK, Griffin BP, Miklaszewska JM, et al: Tegretol (carbamazepine): a controlled trial of a new anti-convulsant. Br J Psychiatry 112:737–742, 1966

Blumer D, Heilbronn M, Himmelhoch J: Indications for carbamazepine in mental illness: atypical psychiatric disorder or temporal lobe epilepsy. Compr Psychiatry 29:108–122, 1988

Browne TR: Valproic acid. N Engl J Med 302:661–666, 1980

Buck OD, Havey P: Combined carbamazepine and lithium therapy for violent behavior (letter). Am J Psychiatry 143:1487, 1986

Choonara IA: Sodium valproate and enuresis (letter). Lancet 1:1276, 1985

Chouinard G: Clonazepam in the treatment of psychiatric disorders, in Use of Anticonvulsants in Psychiatry. Edited by McElroy SL, Pope HG Jr. Clifton, NJ, Oxford Health Care, 1988, pp 43–58

Crosley CJ, Swender PT: Dystonia associated with carbamazepine administration: experience in brain-damaged children. Pediatrics 63:612–615, 1979

D'Hollander L: Traitment au Moyen de Carbamazepine de l'Epilepsi Avec Troubles du Comportement Chez des Enfants Arrierees Mentales en Institut Medicopedagogique. Acta Psychiatr Belg 79:557–569, 1979

Dalby MA: Behavioral effects of carbamazepine, in Advances in Neurology, Vol 11. Edited by Penry JK, Daly DD. New York, Raven, 1975, pp 331–343

Devinsky O, Bear D: Varieties of aggressive behavior in temporal lobe epilepsy. Am J Psychiatry 141:651–656, 1984

Donner M, Frisk M: Carbamazepine treatment of epileptic and psychic symptoms in children and adolescents. Ann Paediat Fenn 11:91–97, 1965

Franks RD, Richter AJ: Schizophrenia-like psychosis associated with anticonvulsant toxicity. Am J Psychiatry 136:973–974, 1979

Freinhar JP: Clonazepam treatment of a mentally retarded woman (letter). Am J Psychiatry 143:1513, 1985

Gay PE: Effects of antiepileptic drugs and seizure type on operant responding in mentally retarded persons. Epilepsia 25:377–386, 1984

Gedye A: Extreme self-injury attributed to frontal lobe seizures. Am J Ment Retard 94:20–26, 1989a

Gedye A: Episodic rage and aggression attributed to frontal lobe seizures. J Ment Defic Res 33:369–380, 1989b

Glue P: Rapid cycling affective disorders in the mentally retarded. Biol Psychiatry 26:250–256, 1989

Greenblatt DJ, Miller LG, Shader RI: Clonazepam pharmacokinetics, brain uptake, and receptor interactions. J Clin Psychiatry 48 (suppl 10):4–9, 1987

Gupta BK, Fish DN, Yerevanian BI: Carbamazepine for intermittent explosive disorder in a Prader-Willi syndrome patient (letter). J Clin Psychiatry 48:423, 1987

Himmelhoch JM: Major mood disorders related to epileptic changes, in Psychiatric Aspects of Epilepsy. Edited by Blumer D. Washington, DC, American Psychiatric Press, 1984, pp 271–294

Itil TM, Soldatos C: Epileptogenic side effects of psychotropic drugs. JAMA 244:1460–1463, 1980

Joffe RT, Post RM, Roy-Byrne PP, et al: Hematological effects of carbamazepine in patients with affective illness. Am J Psychiatry 142:1196–1199, 1985

Kanjilal DC: An evaluation of Tegretol in adults with epilepsy, in Tegretol in Epilepsy: Proceedings of an International Meeting. Edited by Roberts FD. London, Geigy Pharmaceuticals, 1977, pp 55–57

Langee HR: A retrospective study of mentally retarded patients with behavioral disorders who were treated with carbamazepine. Am J Ment Retard 93:640–643, 1989

Marin DB, Greenwald BS: Carbamazepine for aggressive agitation in demented patients during nursing care (letter). Am J Psychiatry 6:805, 1989

McAllister TW: Carbamazepine in mixed frontal lobe and psychiatric disorders. J Clin Psychiatry 46:393–394, 1985

McAllister TW, Price TRP: Aspects of behavior of psychiatric inpatients with frontal lobe damage: some implications for diagnosis and treatment. Compr Psychiatry 28:14–21, 1987

McCracken JT, Diamond RP: Bipolar disorder in mentally retarded adolescents. J Am Acad Child Adol Psychiatry 27:494–499, 1988

McElroy SL, Pope HG Jr (eds): Use of Anticonvulsants in Psychiatry. Clifton, NJ, Oxford Health Care, 1988

McElroy SL, Keck PE Jr, Pope HG Jr, et al: Valproate in the treatment of rapid-cycling bipolar disorder. J Clin Psychopharmacol 8:275–279, 1988a

McElroy SL, Keck PE Jr, Pope HG Jr, et al: Valproate in primary psychiatric disorders: literature review and clinical experience in a private psychiatric hospital, in Use of Anticonvulsants in Psychiatry. Edited by McElroy SL, Pope HG Jr. Clifton, NJ, Oxford Health Care, 1988b, pp 25–41

McQuiston HL, Adler LA, Leong S: Carbamazepine in frontal lobe syndrome: two more cases (letter). J Clin Psychiatry 48:456, 1987

Myers WC, Carrera F: Carbamazepine-induced mania with hypersexuality in a 9-year-old boy (letter). Am J Psychiatry 146:400, 1989

Naylor GJ, Donald JM, Le Poidevin D, et al: A double blind trial of long-term lithium therapy in mental defectives. Br J Psychiatry 124:52–57, 1974

Nurnberger GJ Jr, Guroff JJ, Hamovit J, et al: A family study of rapid-cycling bipolar illness. J Affective Disord 15:87–99, 1988

Panayiotopoulos CP: Nocturnal enuresis associated with sodium valproate. Lancet 1:980–981, 1985

Papez JW: A proposed mechanism of emotion. Arch Neurol Psychiatry 27:725–743, 1937

Patterson JF: Carbamazepine for assaultive patients with organic brain disease. Psychosomatics 28:579–581, 1987

Pleak RR, Birmaher B, Gavrilescu A, et al: Mania and neuropsychiatric excitation following carbamazepine. J Am Acad Child Adol Psychiatry 27:500–503, 1988

Pollack MH, Rosenbaum JF: Management of antidepressant-induced side-effects: a practical guide for the clinician. J Clin Psychiatry 48:3–8, 1987

Post RM: Time course of clinical effects of carbamazepine: implications for mechanisms of action. J Clin Psychiatry 49 (suppl 4):35–46, 1988

Post RM, Uhde TW: Carbamazepine in bipolar illness. Psychopharmacol Bull 21:10–17, 1985

Post RM, Uhde TW, Roy-Byrne PP: Antidepressant effects of carbamazepine. Am J Psychiatry 143:29–34, 1986

Post RM, Kramlinger KG, Uhde TW: Carbamazepine-lithium combination: clinical efficacy and side effects. Int Drug Ther Newslett 22:5–8, 1987

Rapport MD, Sonis WA, Fialkov MJ, et al: Carbamazepine and behavior therapy for aggressive behavior. Behav Modification 7:255–265, 1983

Ratey JJ, Mikkelsen E, Sorgi P, et al: The treatment of aggressive behaviors. J Clin Psychopharmacol 7:35–41, 1987

Ratey JJ, Sovner R, Mikkelsen E, et al: Buspirone therapy for maladaptive behavior and anxiety in developmentally disabled persons. J Clin Psychiatry 50:382–384, 1989

Reid AH: Psychoses in adult mental defectives, I: manic depressive psychosis. Br J Psychiatry 120:205–212, 1972

Reid AH, Ballinger BR, Heather BB: Behavioral syndromes identified by cluster analysis in a sample of 100 severely and profoundly retarded adults. Psychol Med 8:399–412, 1978

Reid AH, Naylor GJ, Kay DSS: A double-blind, placebo controlled crossover trial of carbamazepine in overactive severely mentally handicapped patients. Psychol Med 11:109–113, 1981

Reid AH, Ballinger BR, Heather BB, et al: The natural history of behavioral symptoms among severely and profoundly mentally retarded patients. Br J Psychiatry 145:289–293, 1984

Richardson SA, Koller H, Katz M: Seizures and epilepsy in a mentally retarded population over the first 22 years of life. Appl Res Ment Retard 1:123–138, 1980

Rivinus T: Psychiatric effects of the anticonvulsant regimens. J Clin Psychopharmacol 2:165–192, 1982

Roberts JKA: Neuropsychiatric complications of mental retardation. Psychiatr Clin North Am 9:647–657, 1986

Ross ED, Stewart RS: Pathological display of affect in patients with depression and right frontal brain damage. J Nerv Ment Dis 175:165–172, 1987

Schou M: Lithium prophylaxis: myths and realities. Am J Psychiatry 146:573–576, 1989

Shukla S, Godwin CD, Long LEB, et al: Lithium-carbamazepine neurotoxicity and risk factors. Am J Psychiatry 141:1604–1606, 1984

Signer SF, Benson DF, Rudnick FD: Undetected affective disorder in the developmentally retarded (letter). Am J Psychiatry 143:259, 1986

Silverstein FS, Parrish MA, Johnston MV: Adverse behavioral reactions in children treated with carbamazepine (Tegretol). J Pediatr 101:785–787, 1982

Simpson DM, Foster D: Improvement in organically disturbed behavior with trazodone treatment. J Clin Psychiatry 47:191–193, 1986

Slater E, Roth M: Mayer-Gross Slater and Roth Clinical Psychiatry, 3rd Edition. Baltimore, MD, Williams & Wilkins, 1969

Sovner R: Limiting factors in the use of DSM-III criteria with mentally ill/mentally retarded persons. Psychopharmacol Bull 22:1055–1059, 1986

Sovner R: Anticonvulsant drug therapy of neuropsychiatric disorders in mentally retarded persons, in Use of Anticonvulsants in Psychiatry. Edited by McElroy SL, Pope HG Jr. Clifton, NJ, Oxford Health Care, 1988a, pp 169–181

Sovner R: Behavioral psychopharmacology, in Mental Retardation and Mental Health: Classification, Diagnosis, Treatment, Services. Edited by Stark J, Menolascino FJ, Albarielli M, Gray V. New York, Springer-Verlag, 1988b, pp 229–242

Sovner R: A clinically significant interaction between carbamazepine and valproic acid. J Clin Psychopharmacol 8:448–449, 1988c

Sovner R: Developments in the use of psychotropic drugs. Current Opinion in Psychiatry 2:636–640, 1989a

Sovner R: The use of valproate in the treatment of mentally retarded persons with typical and atypical bipolar disorders. J Clin Psychiatry 50 (suppl 3):40–43, 1989b

Sovner R, Hurley AD: Do the mentally retarded suffer from affective illness? Arch Gen Psychiatry 40:61–67, 1983

Sovner R, Pary RJ: Affective disorders in developmentally disabled persons, in Psychopathology in the Mentally Retarded, 2nd Edition. Edited by Matson JL, Barrett RP. San Antonio, TX, Psychological Association (in press)

Vining EPG, Mellits ED, Dorsen MM, et al: Psychologic and behavioral effects of antiepileptic drugs in children: a double-blind comparison between phenobarbital and valproic acid. Pediatrics 80:165–174, 1987

Wehr TA, Goodwin FK: Can antidepressants cause mania and worsen the course of affective illness? Am J Psychiatry 144:1403–1411, 1987

Williams CA, Tiefenback S, McReynolds JW: Valproic acid-induced hyperammonemia in mentally retarded adults. Neurology 34:550–553, 1984

Chapter 6

Effects of Opioid Receptor Antagonists in the Treatment of Autism and Self-injurious Behavior

Barbara H. Herman, Ph.D.

D uring the past 5 years, there has been a rapid accumulation of research that has suggested a role for opioid peptides in the biochemical etiology of autism and self-injurious behavior (SIB) (Barrett et al. 1989; Bernstein et al. 1987; Campbell et al. 1988a, 1989; Davidson et al. 1983; Gillberg et al. 1985; Herman et al. 1985, 1986, 1987, 1988a, 1989a; Leboyer et al. 1988; Richardson and Zaleski 1983; Ross et al. 1987; Sandman 1988; Sandman et al. 1983, 1987; Sandyk 1985; Weizman et al. 1984, 1988; Zelnik et al. 1986), and reviews of some of this research along with the development of novel opioid autism and SIB hypotheses have been summarized by our laboratory as well as other researchers (Chamberlain and Herman 1990; Deutsch 1986; Herman 1990; Kalat 1978; Panksepp 1979; Panksepp and Sahley 1987; Panksepp et al. 1978a, 1980a, 1980b). More recently, Herman et al. (1988a) elaborated further on this hypothesis and proposed that a subgroup of autistic and SIB individuals may have a dysregulation in proopiomelanocortin (POMC) systems of the hypothalamic-pituitary-adrenal (HPA) axis. This proposal is based on some of the research implicating the potent POMC opioid peptide, β-endorphin (β-E) in autism and SIB (Herman 1990; Herman et al. 1988a; Ross et al. 1987; Sandman 1988; Weizman et al. 1984, 1988; Zelnik et al. 1986), and other investigations implicating nonopioid POMC peptides, such as adrenocorticotropic hormone (ACTH) or the related nonopioid POMC peptide, cortisol, in autism and SIB (Herman 1990; Herman et al. 1986, 1988a; Hoshino et al. 1984, 1987; Jensen et al. 1985).

The POMC autism/SIB hypothesis does not exclude the possibility that other neurochemical systems are involved in autism and SIB. Indeed, there is evidence for etiologic roles for serotonin (5-hydroxytryptamine [5-HT]) in autism (Anderson et al. 1987; Campbell et al.

107

1975, 1986a, 1986b; Hanley et al. 1977; Ritvo et al. 1970, 1983, 1984, 1986; Schain and Freedman 1961; Takahashi et al. 1976; Todd and Ciaranello 1985; Young et al. 1982; Yuwiler and Freedman 1987; Yuwiler et al. 1971, 1975), dopamine (DA) in autism (Anderson et al. 1984; Cohen et al. 1977; Gillberg et al. 1983), and norepinephrine (NE) in SIB (Ratey et al. 1986, 1987). Several excellent reviews present the evidence for a relationship between indolamines and catecholamines in autism and SIB (Aman et al. 1985; Campbell 1988; Campbell and Spencer 1988; Campbell et al. 1981, 1987a; Cataldo and Harris 1982; Du Verglas et al. 1988; Singh and Millichamp 1985).

Advances in neurobiology, such as findings of multiple neurotransmitters in a single neuronal cell body (Lundberg and Hokfelt 1983), argue that simplistic models of brain-based disorders emphasizing a single neurochemical system in that disorder are doomed to failure, since these models do not incorporate the neurochemical complexity of the basic element of the brain—the neuron. On the other hand, it has been shown for several different psychiatric disorders, such as schizophrenia and depression, that a particular class of drugs can be uniquely efficacious in the treatment of a significant portion of individuals with that disorder (Snyder 1984). Since some of these drugs show a striking degree of neurochemical or neuroreceptor specificity, there is indirect evidence that a single neurochemical or neuroreceptor system may be of fundamental importance in the etiology of a psychiatric disorder. The neurochemical complexity of these psychiatric disorders is made obvious by treatment failures in some individuals with seemingly the same psychiatric disorder and the incomplete effectiveness of some of the drug treatments. With these cautions in mind (concerning simplistic neurochemical models of psychiatric disorders), my aim in this chapter is to review preclinical and clinical research implicating opioid peptides and the POMC system in autism and SIB. A detailed analysis of DA, 5-HT, and NE systems is excluded so that I may focus in greater depth on the opioid and POMC systems. At the conclusion of the chapter, I present a novel model that predicts a link between POMC and 5-HT dysfunctions of the brain in autism (Chamberlain and Herman 1990).

OPIOID AND POMC SYSTEMS OF THE BRAIN AND PITUITARY

Opioids are endogenous peptides that act like morphine in the central nervous system (CNS) (for review, see Akil et al. 1984; Cox 1982;

Goldstein 1984; Khachaturian et al. 1985; Mansour et al. 1988; O'Donohue and Dorsa 1982; Watson et al. 1977). There are three major groups of opioid peptides derived from larger precursor hormones with genetically distinct origins: POMC, from which β-E and fragments of β-E are derived; preproenkephalin, from which Met-enkephalin, Leu-enkephalin, and seven other opioids are derived; preprodynorphin, from which dynorphin and neoendorphin peptides are derived.

The POMC system consists primarily of cell bodies in the intermediate and anterior lobes of the pituitary and in the arcuate nucleus of the hypothalamus, which project long axons to diverse subcortical regions of the brain, including the limbic ("emotional") brain (O'Donohue and Dorsa 1982; Watson et al. 1977). There is also a small cluster of POMC cell bodies in the nucleus tractus solitarius of the brain stem (Khachaturian et al. 1985). POMC cell bodies release multiple neuromodulators including β-lipotropin, the opioid peptide, β-E, ACTH, corticotropinlike intermediate peptide, and forms of melanocyte-stimulating hormone. Thus, several neuromodulators are produced from one large precursor hormone by enzymatic cleavage at specific amino acid sites of POMC. Plasma β-E is believed to originate almost exclusively from the pituitary, since hypophysectomy results in nearly a complete depletion of immunoreactive β-E concentrations in rats (Guillemin et al. 1977; Houghton et al. 1980) and humans (Schlachter et al. 1983). On the other hand, cerebrospinal fluid (CSF) and brain immunoreactive β-E appears to come from brain POMC cell bodies, since hypophysectomy does not influence brain immunoreactive β-E concentrations in rats (Houghton et al. 1980; Rossier et al. 1977) and only partially decreases CSF concentrations in humans. These POMC hormone products have been individually implicated in various emotional and psychiatric processes in adults (Gispen-DeWied et al. 1987) and have recently been linked to pediatric psychiatric disorders, such as autism (Campbell et al. 1988a; Herman et al. 1986; LeBoyer et al. 1988; Ross et al. 1987) and SIB (Barrett et al. 1989; Herman et al. 1987; Sandyk 1985). β-endorphin is of particular interest, since it is an opioid peptide that is about 100 times more potent than morphine as an analgesic (Herman et al. 1980) and may have a significant influence on human affect. Finally, there are multiple types of opioid receptors in the CNS, including μ, δ, and κ types, to which the opioid peptides show dramatically different affinities. Thus, the opioid peptide systems of the brain are complex families of chemicals that offer a diversity of neuromodulators and receptors that may influence myriad CNS functions.

OPIOID AND POMC HYPOTHESES OF AUTISM AND SIB

Opioid Autism Hypothesis

Panksepp (1979) proposed that autism is caused by a failure of striatal β-E to diminish with maturation. This hypothesis represents a refinement of an earlier proposal that heightened activity in some brain opioid system may underlie autism (Herman and Panksepp 1978; Panksepp et al. 1978a, 1978b), a construct that was also suggested by Kalat (1978) and Deutsch (1986). This would explain why separation-distress responses are typically reduced in autistic children (Herman et al. 1986; Kanner 1943; although see Sigman and Mundy 1989); that is, the separation-distress system is inhibited by increased tone in some central opioid pathway (Herman and Panksepp 1978, 1981; Panksepp et al. 1978a, 1978b). Therefore, social attachments may not be necessary for autistic children, since they may derive a similar type of reinforcement from their own opioid systems.

Opioid SIB Hypothesis

Herman et al. (1987) proposed that enhanced brain opioid activity may underlie SIB, especially given the evidence linking opioids and antinociception (Adams 1976; Herman et al. 1980). In healthy individuals, pain-producing behavior stops quickly. In self-injurious individuals, SIB may not induce pain, since these individuals may be in an opioid analgesic state. Accordingly, there may be little motivation to terminate SIB. Although this hypothesis is capable of explaining why certain individuals may not terminate SIB, it does not explain why an individual would initiate the behavior.

A second hypothesis that explains the motivation for SIB is one described by Cataldo and Harris (1982), proposing that individuals may engage in SIB as a method to self-administer endogenous opioids. Indeed, rats will self-administer opioids (e.g., enkephalins) directly into the ventricles of their brains (Belluzzi and Stein 1977). In addition, individuals engaging in a long-distance run (e.g., a 100-mile race) have been reported to show elevations in plasma immunoreactive β-E concentrations (Bortz et al. 1981). At this time, however, there is no evidence that opioids are released as a consequence of SIB, and these studies are associated with extremely difficult methodological problems.

POMC Autism/SIB Hypothesis

I have presented a novel biochemical model for autism and SIB, which proposes that a subgroup of individuals with these disorders may have a hypersecretion of pineal melatonin that produces a cascade of biochemical effects, including a corresponding hyposecretion of pituitary POMC peptides (e.g., β-E and ACTH) and a hypersecretion of hypothalamic β-E and 5-HT (Figure 6-1; Chamberlain and Herman 1990; Herman et al. 1988a). This model is described in detail at the end of this chapter. In brief, one of the strongest lines of evidence to support this model is the results of an investigation indicating that about 60% of non-self-injurious autistic and SIB children show an abnormal blunted plasma immunoreactive β-E, immunoreactive ACTH, and a cortisol response to naltrexone (Herman 1990; Herman et al. 1988a; B.H. Herman, A. Arthur-Smith, K. Verebey, J. Alrazi, M.K. Hammock, 1989, unpublished observations). This and other lines of evidence supporting this hypothesis are reviewed in detail in this chapter.

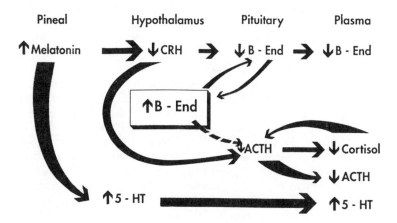

Figure 6-1. Biochemical model linking dysfunctions in brain melatonin, proopiomelanocortin peptides, and serotonin in autism. Hypersecretion of melatonin is proposed to induce hyperserotonemia in brain and blood. Increased production of pineal melatonin is also proposed to inhibit release of hypothalamic corticotropin-releasing hormone (CRH). Decreased CRH results in decreased release of pituitary β-endorphin (β-E) and adrenocorticotropic hormone (ACTH). This, in turn, would be expected to result in decreased plasma concentrations of β-E, ACTH, and cortisol. It is proposed that autistic individuals have genetically determined hypersecretion of hypothalamic β-E, which may further contribute to inhibition of pituitary and plasma β-E (Chamberlain and Herman 1990; Herman et al. 1988a). B-End, β-endorphin; 5-HT, 5-hydroxytryptamine. Reprinted with permission from Chamberlain and Herman (1990).

PRECLINICAL EVIDENCE FOR ROLE OF OPIOIDS IN AUTISM AND SIB

Opioids and Social Attachment in Animals

One of the most pronounced dysfunctions observed in autistic individuals is impaired social attachment or interaction (DSM-III-R, American Psychiatric Association 1987). This abnormality may be a major obstacle preventing autistic individuals from developing normal communicative skills (Akerly 1974). Because an important component of autism is a qualitative impairment in verbal communication (DSM-III-R), it is doubtful that any animal model will fully duplicate this disorder. Attempts have been made, however, to study discrete aspects of some of the social abnormalities associated with autism. Since social attachment is a drive that exists in numerous animal species from rats to humans, it is conceivable that studies focusing on the biology of attachment may be relevant to the social deficits in autism. An excellent review of such animal behavioral studies was provided by Panksepp and Sahley (1987), and here I only briefly summarize the major lines of animal behavioral research that support the opioid autism hypothesis.

The opioid autism hypothesis was derived from animal research suggesting that there is an important relationship between brain opioid systems and social attachment in infant animals (Herman and Panksepp 1978, 1981; Panksepp 1979; Panksepp and DeEskinazi 1980; Panksepp et al. 1978a, 1978b, 1978c, 1980a, 1980b). Responses occurring during acute maternal separation are one of the primary methods for measuring social attachment in children (Bell and Ainsworth 1972; Bowlby 1969) and animals (Harlow 1958; Herman and Panksepp 1978). One measure of separation distress is the distress vocalization (DV) or crying that infants exhibit when involuntarily separated from their mothers. Low doses of morphine (less than 1 mg/kg sc) induce dose-dependent decreases in separation DV in infant rhesus monkeys, dogs, guinea pigs, and chickens (Herman and Panksepp 1978; Kalin and Shelton 1989; Panksepp et al. 1978a, 1978b, 1980b). These doses are an order of magnitude below the dose required to induce analgesia, suggesting that brain areas modulating separation distress are extremely sensitive to opioids. In addition, naloxone (a specific opiate antagonist) increases the frequency of separation DV in infant animals (Herman and Panksepp 1978; Kalin and Shelton 1989; Panksepp et al. 1978a, 1978b, 1978c). These data indicate that brain opioids inhibit separation distress and that naloxone exacerbates distress by blocking endogenous opioids. Subsequent research (Herman and Panksepp 1981) showed where in the brain these DV areas were localized and once again indicated that these systems interfaced with opioid pathways in the brain. A second measure of social attachment is the maintenance of proximity by an infant to its primary caretaker (Bowlby 1969; Harlow 1958; Herman and Panksepp 1978). In animals, morphine decreases infant-maternal proximity maintenance time (Herman and Panksepp 1978) and other social behaviors (Panksepp and DeEskinazi 1980). Morphine may decrease approach attachment by replacing the function normally subserved by opioids in the reinforcement of social bonds (Herman and Panksepp 1978). These investigations suggest a role for brain opioid peptides in social attachment and, by extension, suggest that aberrations in attachment may reflect dysfunctions in opioids.

Opioid Model of SIB in Animals

In the early 1980s, I investigated the cross-tolerance between the highly selective μ opioid receptor agonist, sufentanil, and the κ receptor ligand, dynorphin-(1-13), in rats (Herman and Goldstein 1981). Sufentanil is an extremely potent opiate that is about 1,000 to 10,000 times more potent as an analgesic than morphine. The goal of our study was to make brain μ opioid receptors tolerant by repeated systemic subcutaneous administration of sufentanil and then to determine whether the rats showed cross-tolerance to dynorphin. The dependent measure was opioid-induced catalepsy. The procedure to make the rats tolerant involved repeated injections of high doses of sufentanil throughout an 8-hour period. Rats that had received systemic sufentanil showed complete cross-tolerance (i.e., no catalepsy) in response to intraventricularly administered sufentanil. In contrast, sufentanil-tolerant rats showed a greatly reduced effect to intraventricular dynorphin-(1-13), confirming that the dynorphin cataleptic effect was not mediated by a μ opioid receptor. A disturbing effect emerged during the study. Many of the sufentanil-treated rats gnawed off the digits of their forepaws and hindpaws. These same rats were also observed to engage in frequent nonnutritive gnawing behavior (e.g., gnawing the floor of the individual Plexiglas cages in which they were housed). My initial concern was to minimize this SIB by physically intervening (when possible) when a rat began to gnaw off its digits. I also realized that a second experiment had just been conducted. The results of this experiment indicated that a μ opioid receptor agonist could induce SIB, and these findings supported the notion that heightened opioid activity in the brain may underlie SIB. I soon realized that this was not a novel scientific observation, since

Carroll and Lim (1960) had discovered that chronic high doses of morphine induced SIB in rats. In any case, results of these studies indicated that chronic high doses of μ opioid receptors agonists in rats could serve as a pharmacological model for SIB. Obviously, additional investigations using the sufentanil- or morphine-SIB model are needed to determine the parameters of this effect and to address more specific questions about biochemical and neuroanatomical organization for this effect.

CLINICAL BIOCHEMICAL EVIDENCE FOR ROLE OF POMC PEPTIDES IN AUTISM AND SIB

Opioids in CSF and Plasma of Autistic Children

Studies of opioid concentrations in the plasma and CSF of autistic individuals have provided data in support of an opioid hypothesis of autism, and I present a summary of these data in Table 6-1. Gillberg et al. (1985) and Ross et al. (1987) independently reported elevated opioid peptide CSF concentrations in autistic children compared with sex- and age-matched control subjects. In both cases, opioid CSF concentrations were about twofold higher in autistic subjects compared with control subjects, although Gillberg et al. (1985) measured Fraction II opioids whereas Ross et al. (1987) measured immunoreactive β-E concentrations. In addition, results of the Ross et al. (1987) study suggested that the serotonin-depleting drug, fenfluramine, reduced CSF immunoreactive β-E concentrations, although this effect failed to reach a conventional level of significance. This finding is of note, since the biochemical model that I describe at the end of this chapter predicts an interaction between 5-HT and opioid systems in autism.

Weizman et al. (1984) found that plasma humoral endorphin was significantly reduced in autistic children by about 27% compared with control subjects. Our laboratory has failed to find any significant differences in immunoreactive β-E plasma concentrations in non-self-injurious autistic children compared with control subjects, although there was a trend for the autistic children to have slightly lower levels (Herman et al. 1986, 1988a). Weizman et al. (1988) indicated that plasma immunoreactive β-E concentrations of unmedicated autistic subjects were significantly lower (by about 50%) compared with age- and sex-matched unmedicated schizophrenic patients and healthy control subjects. Many of the autistic subjects in the Weizman et al. (1984, 1988) studies were self-injurious (R. Weizman, September 24, 1988, personal communication), unlike the autistic subjects in the Herman et al. (1986) study. A comparison of the values in Table 6-1

Table 6-1. Concentrations of opioid peptides in cerebrospinal fluid and plasma of autistic, self-injurious, and control subjects

Opioid	Source	Concentration		Ratio[b]	Reference
		Autistic[a]	Control		
β-E	CSF	16.1 ± 4.4 (9)	9.3 ± 2.3 (9)	H	Ross et al. (1987)
Fraction II	CSF	13,000 ± 2,000 (20)	5,600 ± 800 (8)	H	Gillberg et al. (1985)
β-E	Plasma	6.5 ± 1.0 (5)	7.3 ± .7 (28)	O	Herman et al. (1986)
β-E	Plasma	4.1 ± .3 (8)[c]	8.2 ± 1.1 (8)	L	Weizman et al. (1988)
Hum E	Plasma	827 ± 103 (10)	1,121 ± 75 (11)	L	Weizman et al. (1984)
		Self-injurious[d]	Control		
β-E	Plasma	4.1 ± .5 (3)	8.4 ± 1.5 (10)	L	Zelnik et al. (1986)
β-E	Plasma	4.4 ± .6 (7)	6.8 ± .5 (36)	L	Herman et al. (1988a, 1988b)
β-E	Plasma	9.2(29)[e]	6.5(11)[e]	H	Sandman (1988)

Note. Values are means ± standard errors, with number of subjects in parentheses. Concentrations are expressed as pmol/L, except values for humoral endorphin (Hum E). β-E, β-endorphin. CSF, cerebrospinal fluid. H, opioids higher in autistic or self-injurious subjects than in normal controls. O, no difference in opioids in autistic or self-injurious subjects than in normal controls. L, opioids lower in autistic or self-injurious subjects than in normal controls.

[a] Non-self-injurious autistic children and adolescents.

[b] Concentration of opioids in autistic subjects relative to normal controls or in self-injurious subjects relative to normal controls.

[c] Some of these subjects were also self-injurious.

[d] Self-injurious subjects may or may not be autistic. All are children or adolescents except for those in Sandman (1988) study.

[e] Standard errors not reported.

suggests that the key variable in reduced plasma immunoreactive β-E concentrations of autistic subjects may be SIB. I hypothesize that these seemingly incongruous results for CSF immunoreactive β-E compared with plasma immunoreactive β-E may reflect negative feedback between the hypothalamus and pituitary in the regulation of β-E in the brain and plasma, respectively (Zelnik et al. 1986). The β-E negative feedback hypothesis developed in 1986 (Zelink et al. 1986) has been incorporated in the POMC autism model presented in Figure 6-1.

Opioids in CSF and Plasma of SIB Children

There have been a few reports on the concentrations of opioid peptides in the plasma and CSF of children exhibiting SIB. This is relevant to autism, since some autistic individuals exhibit SIB (Coleman and Gillberg 1985). In 1986, my laboratory reported that plasma immunoreactive β-E concentrations were significantly lower in three SIB male children (mean ± standard error 4.10 ± .49 pmol/L compared with 10 age-matched male control subjects (8.37 ± 1.46 pmol/L) (Zelnik et al. 1986). More recently, my group has obtained similar results for plasma immunoreactive β-E concentrations in a larger sample of subjects involving seven SIB male children (4.40 ± .60 pmol/L) compared with 36 age-matched male control subjects (6.85 ± .46 pmol/L) (Herman 1990; Herman et al. 1988a, 1988b). These findings are particularly convincing, since the subjects in the studies were extremely self-injurious (≥35 SIB attempts per 5-minute test session) and the results were not confounded by possible effects of concurrent pharmacotherapies on plasma immunoreactive β-E concentrations (i.e., each subject was free of drugs for at least 4 weeks before obtaining those samples). These results are similar to those of Weizman et al. (1984, 1988) for plasma humoral endorphin immunoreactive β-E concentrations in autistic children. In contrast, Sandman (1988) reported that plasma immunoreactive β-E concentrations are significantly higher by about 29% in institutionalized mentally retarded adult individuals with SIB compared with sex- and age-matched institutionalized mentally retarded control subjects without SIB. The discrepancy between the studies is unexplained but may be related to the age of the subjects sampled, concurrent drug treatment, institutionalization, or radioimmunoassay. It is interesting that the difference between these studies appears to be in the values for the SIB subjects and not the control subjects (see Table 6-1), possibly ruling out institutionalization as a factor. There is evidence that opioid peptides are greatly elevated in the CSF of certain SIB individuals. For example, Gillberg et al. (1985) found that a majority of SIB children (9 of 12) have concentrations of Fraction II opioids that are severalfold higher than those found in children without SIB (3 of 12). These data suggest that a negative-feedback relationship in the regulation of β-E in CSF and plasma may exist in SIB individuals, which is similar to that described for autistic individuals. In addition, these data indicate that future studies measuring immunoreactive β-E concentrations of autistic individuals should conduct separate analyses of the significance of concurrent SIB and non-SIB within autistic subjects.

Nonopioid POMC Peptides in Autism

Little research has been reported on the other nonopioid POMC bioactive peptides, with the possible exception of cortisol, which is regulated by the POMC peptide ACTH. For example, Herman et al. (1988a, 1988b) reported that non-SIB autistic children ($N = 5$, 250 ± 42 nmol/L) have significantly lower plasma cortisol concentrations than sex- and age-matched control subjects ($N = 8$, 374 ± 7 nmol/L). Based on this finding, a similar hyposecretion in plasma ACTH concentrations may be found in autistic subjects, and my colleagues and I are currently examining this question in our laboratory.

Use of Dexamethasone and Naltrexone to Assess Biochemical Status of POMC HPA Axis

Further evidence for cortisol HPA axis disturbance in autism is provided by two studies by Hoshino et al. (1984, 1987), indicating that some autistic children show an abnormal diurnal rhythm or dexamethasone suppression test (DST) for saliva cortisol. These HPA axis disturbances were more common in low-functioning autistic subjects than in high-functioning autistic subjects. In the 1984 study, Hoshino et al. conducted DSTs in 19 autistic children, 26 healthy volunteers, 19 schizophrenic patients, and 15 children with mental retardation (MR) or minimal brain dysfunction (MBD). All healthy and schizophrenic subjects, all MBD children ($N = 5$), and 9 of 10 MR children showed DST cortisol suppression (a normal response). In contrast, none of the 8 low-functioning autistic subjects and 9 of the 11 high-functioning autistic subjects showed suppression. Similarly, Jensen et al. (1985) reported that 11 of 13 autistic children failed to show plasma cortisol suppression in response to DST. Hoshino et al. (1984, 1987) proposed that the negative-feedback mechanism of the HPA axis may be disturbed in low-functioning autistic subjects because of the dysfunctions in 5-HT metabolism in this population. Independent of Hoshino, I had proposed a disturbance in the HPA axis in autistic and SIB children, and this served as the motivation in our laboratory for collecting plasma samples for ACTH and cortisol in autistic and SIB children first presented in 1986 (e.g., Herman et al. 1986; Zelnik et al. 1986). This concept of an HPA axis disturbance in autism has been incorporated in the POMC autism model presented in Figure 6-1.

Herman et al. (1988a) reported abnormalities in the plasma cortisol, immunoreactive β-E, and immunoreactive ACTH response of autistic children to naltrexone. The response of healthy adults to naltrexone is about a twofold elevation in plasma cortisol, immunoreactive β-E, and immunoreactive ACTH concentrations (Blankstein et al. 1980; Delitala et al. 1981; Judd et al. 1981; Kosten et al. 1986; Mendelson et al. 1986; Morley et al. 1980; Pomara et al. 1988). Thus, in healthy individuals, opioid receptors blockade results

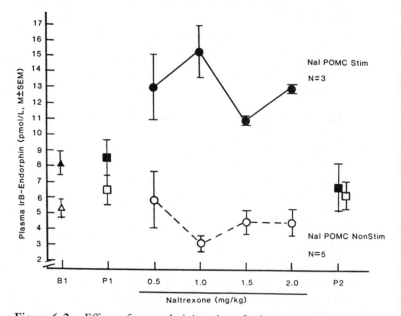

Figure 6-2. Effects of acute administration of naltrexone (.5, 1.0, 1.5, and 2.0 mg/kg) compared with placebo (P1, P2) on plasma concentrations of immunoreactive β-endorphin (β-E) in eight non-self-injurious autistic children. Three subjects showed more than twofold increases in plasma immunoreactive β-E in response to naltrexone (Nal POMC Stim, normal response), and remaining five children failed to show significant effects of naltrexone on plasma immunoreactive β-E (Nal POMC NonStim, abnormal response) (Herman et al. 1988a).

in the increased release of pituitary-derived β-E and ACTH, possibly as a result of feedback inhibition between opioid receptors and the cell bodies of the pituitary that produce POMC peptides. This feedback relationship appears to be dysfunctional in autistic subjects, however. Herman et al. (1988a) found that five of eight autistic subjects (62%) and three of five self-injurious children (60%) failed to show any increase in plasma cortisol and immunoreactive β-E concentrations in response to acute doses of naltrexone (.5, 1.0, 1.5, and 2.0 mg/kg) (Figures 6-2 and 6-3). (Plasma peptide response to naltrexone for self-injurious children is described in detail in Herman 1990.) Each dose of naltrexone produced a minimum of a twofold increase in plasma cortisol and immunoreactive β-E concentrations in the remaining autistic subjects. Similar effects of naltrexone were found on plasma ACTH concentrations. These data suggest that naltrexone may reveal the status of the POMC HPA axis in autism in a manner similar to the DST for depression. Further, results of this

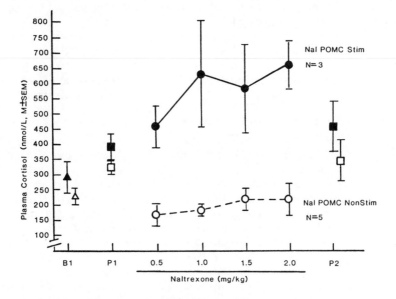

Figure 6-3. Effects of acute administration of naltrexone (.5, 1.0, 1.5, and 2.0 mg/kg) compared with placebo (P1, P2) on plasma concentrations of cortisol in same eight non-self-injurious subjects described in caption to Figure 6-2. Three autistic children who showed twofold increases in plasma immunoreactive β-endorphin in response to naltrexone also showed similar increases in plasma cortisol (Nal POMC Stim) (Herman et al. 1988a).

study provide independent confirmation using a different HPA-stimulating drug of dysfunction of the HPA axis in autism.

PHARMACOLOGICAL EVIDENCE FOR ROLE OF OPIOID PEPTIDES IN AUTISM

Pharmacological Properties of Naltrexone

Naltrexone is a drug that is a relatively pure opiate antagonist (Verebey et al. 1976). Naltrexone has far greater therapeutic usefulness in psychiatry than the opiate antagonist naloxone. First, unlike naloxone, naltrexone retains much of its efficacy when administered orally (Martin et al. 1973). Second, unlike naloxone, which has a relatively short half-life, the duration of action of naltrexone approached 24 hours after moderate oral doses (Martin et al. 1973). Finally, similar to naloxone, naltrexone selectively antagonizes opioid receptors (particularly μ-type receptors) in living human brains, as measured by positron-emission tomography (Lee et al. 1988). The extraordinary longevity of naltrexone in antagonizing brain opioid receptors is indicated by results of the Lee et al. (1988) study suggesting that as many as one-third of μ opioid receptors in living human brains are blocked as long as 1 week after a moderate oral dose of naltrexone. The rationale underlying these naltrexone studies is that if autistic individuals have an overactivity of brain opioids, then opioid receptor blockade should decrease some autistic symptoms.

Possible Side Effects of Naltrexone

Although most studies using adults as subjects indicate that naltrexone has no detectable side effects (Verebey and Mule 1979; Verebey et al. 1976), there are at least two reports suggesting that naltrexone may induce nausea and reduce food intake in former opiate addicts (Hollister et al. 1981; Mendelson et al. 1979). In addition, in situations in which opioids are mobilized, opiate antagonists have been shown to have cardiovascular effects (Holaday and Faden 1978). Possibly the most serious risk of naltrexone is the putative development of reversible liver toxicity in certain adult patients administered chronic high doses of naltrexone. There are two studies using obese adult patients and patients with Alzheimer's disease as subjects that report that naltrexone doses of 300 mg/kg (about 4 mg/kg) induced increases that were subsequently reversible in serum concentrations of the liver enzymes serum glutamic-oxaloacetic transaminase (SGOT) and serum glutamic-pyruvic transaminase (SGPT) (Mitchell et al. 1987; Pfohl et al. 1986). An important criticism of these two studies is that the liver status of the subjects is questionable and may represent a confounding factor. Accordingly, Herman et al. (1989a, 1989b) examined some of the possible side effects of acute administration of naltrexone in their five autistic subjects. This was a phase 1 study in which subjects were tested once per week for 8 weeks as follows: baseline; baseline; placebo; .5, 1.0, 1.5, and 2.0 mg/kg naltrexone; placebo. The effects of naltrexone on auscultated heart rate, systolic blood pressure, axillary body temperature, and body weight were investigated before and about 1 hour after drug administration. In addition, an electrocardiogram was recorded on each child before and about 3 hours after the placebo or 2.0 mg/kg of naltrexone. Electrocardiogram effects were evaluated by comparing heart rate, axis, PR, QRS, and QT. Finally, the serum concentrations of the liver enzymes SGOT and SGPT were measured 24 hours after placebo or naltrexone administration. Naltrexone had no statistically significant effects on any of these measures compared with baseline or placebo levels. Thus, these data and those of Campbell et al. (1988a, 1988b) provide preliminary evidence for the safety of acute administration of doses of ≤ 2.0 mg/kg naltrexone in children, but data from additional subjects are needed to determine the reliability of these results. Possible side effects of chronic naltrexone administration also need to be evaluated.

Effects of Naltrexone in Autism

There have been few published studies on the effects of opiate antagonists in autism (excluding SIB studies), and a summary of these studies is shown in the top half of Table 6-2. Herman et al. (1986) were the first to report on the behavioral effects of naltrexone in five autistic children. This was a Food and Drug Administration–approved phase 1 study in which subjects were tested once per week for 8 weeks with treatments administered as follows: baseline; baseline; placebo; .5, 1.0, 1.5, and 2.0 mg/kg naltrexone; placebo. Five autistic children (4–12 years of age) were evaluated using a structured social playroom test situation (Brain Research Center [BRC] social-proximity test). This is a 10-minute test designed to determine social interactions of a child toward a familiar adult volunteer in a playroom, and performance is also rated on the Behavior Observation Scale (BOS) for autism (Freeman et al. 1978). A parent questionnaire for autism (the BRC Autism Scale) was also used. Subjects were blind to drug, and sessions were videotaped for blind analysis. Naltrexone induced significant decreases in abnormal motor behaviors (hand flapping and body whirling) associated with autism as revealed by the BOS (Freeman et al. 1978) and the parent autism questionnaire. The effects of naltrexone were most pronounced at the 2.0 mg/kg dose

Table 6-2. Effects of opiate antagonists on autism and self-injurious behavior

Drug (mg/kg)	Diagnosis	n	Age	Hyperactivity	Stereotypical behavior	Social approach	SIB	Reference
Naltrexone (.5–2.0)	Autism	5	C	D	D	I/O	N	Herman et al. (1986)
Naltrexone (.5–2.0)	Autism	8	C	D	D	I	N	Campbell et al. (1988a, 1988b)
Naltrexone (1.0–2.0)	Autism	2	C	D	D	I	D	Leboyer et al. (1988)
Naltrexone (.5–2.0)	SIB	3	C	N	N	N	D	Herman et al. (1987)
Naltrexone (.5–2.0)	SIB	1	C	N	N	N	D	Bernstein et al. (1987)
Naltrexone (.5–2.0)	SIB	4	A	O	O	O	D	Sandman (1988)
Naltrexone (1.0–2.0)	SIB	2	A	N	N	N	O	Szymanski et al. (1987)
Naltrexone (1.0)	SIB	1	A	N	N	N	D	Barrett et al. (1989)
Naltrexone (1.0)	SIB	6	C/A	N	N	N	D/O	Kars et al. (1990)
Naloxone	SIB	2	A	N	N	N	D/O	Sandman et al. (1983)
Naloxone	SIB	1	A	N	N	N	D/O	Davidson et al. (1983)
Naloxone	SIB	1	A	N	N	N	D	Richardson and Zaleski (1983)
Naloxone	SIB	1	C	N	N	N	D	Sandyk (1985)
Naloxone	SIB	2	A	N	N	N	O	Beckwith (1986)
Naloxone	SIB	1	A	N	N	N	D	Bernstein et al. (1987)
Naloxone	SIB	1	C	N	N	N	I	Barrett et al. (1989)

Note. Stereotypical behavior includes hand flapping, body whirling, and pacing. Naltrexone was administered acutely, except for Szymanski et al. (1987), Barrett et al. (1989), and Kars et al. (1990) studies. SIB, self-injurious behavior: Most SIB individuals have dual diagnosis of mental retardation. C, child (3–18 years old); A, adult (>18 years old). D, decrease; I, increase; O, no effect; N, not studied.

for both hand flapping (Figure 6-4) and body whirling. Although statistical analysis failed to reveal a significant effect of naltrexone on quantitative measures of gross locomotor activity, a trend toward a decrease with the 2.0 mg/kg dose was suggested. Consistent with a diagnosis of autism, subjects given a placebo spent the least percentage of time in the social-proximity test in the quadrant containing the volunteer (mean 79%) compared with the empty quadrant (the mean ranges from 21% to 51%). This pattern was not significantly altered by naltrexone, suggesting that acute administration of naltrexone did not significantly influence social-proximity behavior. These findings may reflect the difficulties of assessing the effects of an acutely (as opposed to chronically) administered drug on social behavior. A fourfold increase in eye-contact time with the 2.0 mg/kg dose was also suggested, but elevated postdrug placebo eye-contact scores made this effect difficult to evaluate. This postdrug continuance in elevated eye-contact scores may reflect a drug-induced "social learning effect" or may suggest that sufficient naltrexone was still bound

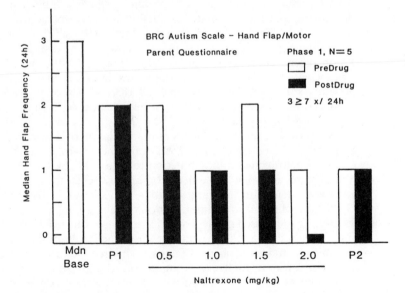

Figure 6-4. Effects of acute administration of naltrexone (.5, 1.0, 1.5, and 2.0 mg/kg) compared with baseline (Mdn) and placebo (P1, P2) on parental ratings of hand-flapping frequency in five non-self-injurious autistic children. PreDrug refers to behavior day before drug; PostDrug refers to behavior on day of drug. Test is BRC autism checklist, with which parents rate frequency of behavior for 24 hours (Herman et al. 1986).

to brain opioid receptors 1 week after drug was administered (Lee et al. 1988). Naltrexone had no significant effect on spontaneous vocalization or the communicative use of language. Overall, the results of this study suggest that acute administration of naltrexone decreased motor stereotypies in a small sample of autistic children.

A second laboratory to investigate the effects of naltrexone in autism was that of Campbell et al. (1988a). This study was an open trial of eight autistic children involving a design similar to that of Herman et al. (1986), and it included the following protocol given during a 6-week period: baseline; baseline; .5, 1.0, and 2.0 mg/kg doses of naltrexone; postdrug sessions. Subjects were eight autistic males (3–6 years of age). Rating scales included the Children's Psychiatric Rating Scale (CPRS), the Clinical Global Impressions (CGI) scale, and Conner's Parent-Teacher Rating Scale (Conner). Using the CPRS, significant improvement was shown with each of the three naltrexone doses for behaviors associated with autism, including social withdrawal, productive speech, and stereotypies. On the CGI scale, one item (severity of illness) showed significant improvement. Total scores on the Conner measure of hyperactivity and conduct disorder showed significant reductions for all three doses. Five of the eight children were reported as showing mild sedation. In a more recent report on this study (Campbell et al. 1989), the sample was increased to 10 autistic children. Results were similar to the previous study and indicated that all three doses of naltrexone produced decreases on the CPRS; administration of .5 mg/kg increased verbal production, and the 2.0 mg/kg dose reduced stereotypies. The only side effect was mild sedation of brief duration. Similar to the Herman et al. (1989a) study, there were no significant effects of naltrexone on liver-function tests (SGOT, SGPT, alkaline phosphatase, and total bilirubin) or on cardiovascular function.

In agreement with the results of these two studies, Leboyer et al. (1988) found that acute administration of naltrexone (1.0, 1.5, and 2.0 mg/kg) decreased the hyperactivity, increased the social behavior, and decreased the SIB of two autistic girls. The results of these three preliminary studies involving 17 autistic children indicate that acute administration of naltrexone decreases the hyperactivity and stereotypy associated with autism and may increase certain social behaviors of autistics.

Effects of Naloxone and Naltrexone on SIB

Numerous laboratories have investigated the effects of the opiate antagonists naloxone and naltrexone on SIB (Table 6-2; for detailed review see Herman 1990). The rationale of these studies is that a pharmacological blockade of brain opioid receptors may lower the pain threshold in these individuals and, in turn, result in a decrease in SIB. Typically, SIB subjects for these studies are mentally retarded, and a small proportion have an additional diagnosis of autism. There are at least three studies suggesting that the short-acting opiate antagonist naloxone decreases SIB. Significant effects of naloxone have been obtained in studies by Sandman et al. (1983, $N = 2$), Bernstein et al. (1987, $N = 1$), and Sandyk (1985, $N = 1$). Results of other naloxone/SIB investigations have suggested mixed results (Davidson et al. 1983, $N = 1$; Richardson and Zaleski 1983, $N = 1$), no effect (Beckwith et al. 1986, $N = 2$), and increases under naloxone (Barrett et al. 1989, $N = 2$). Further, Sandman et al. (1987) reported that naloxone reduced "hallucinatory voices" that instructed an adult female with normal intelligence to engage in SIB. Five more recent investigations have indicated that the long-acting opiate antagonist naltrexone induces significant dose-dependent decreases in the frequency of SIB. The first of these studies was by Herman et al. (1985, 1987, 1989a, 1989b), who reported that naltrexone (.5, 1.0, and 1.5 mg/kg) induced significant decreases in SIB frequency in three males—two who were mentally retarded with autisticlike behaviors (10 and 17 years of age) and one of normal intelligence with Gilles de la Tourette's disease (17 years of age) (Figure 6-5). In a further analysis of these data, Herman et al. (1989b) reported that these inhibitory effects of naltrexone on SIB could be dissociated from effects on heart rate and blood pressure. Sandman (1988) conducted a double-blind, controlled trial of naltrexone (25, 50, and 100 mg) in four mentally retarded adult males. All four subjects showed significant decreases in SIB with naltrexone, but no significant effects of naltrexone were detected on stereotypic behavior, Conner (a hyperactivity rating scale), and the Vineland Adaptive Behavior Scale (a rating scale measuring social behaviors). In a third investigation by Bernstein et al. (1987), naltrexone (50 and 100 mg) significantly decreased SIB frequency in a 15-year-old mentally retarded male. Barrett et al. (1989) reported that naltrexone (50 mg per day) reduced self-injury to near-zero rates in a mentally retarded autistic adolescent. Very recently, Kars and co-workers (1990) utilized a double-blind placebo-controlled design to examine the effects of naltrexone (50 mg daily for 3 consecutive weeks) in six profoundly mentally retarded males (15 to 31 years old). Naltrexone produced significant decreases in SIB frequency in two subjects; one showed a tendency toward reduction, and two no effect. These results parallel those of Herman et al. (1987) indicating the individual variation in response to naltrexone in SIB individuals. To date, the only negative study has been by Szymanski et al. (1987), who reported that naltrexone (50 mg per day and 100 mg per day) had no reliable effects on SIB in two mentally retarded male adults. One possible explanation for Szymanski's et al. (1987) failure to obtain significant effects is that gross clinical observations by a nursing staff were used to assess SIB. In the four positive naltrexone studies, the frequency of SIB was determined during a fixed time period by experienced research raters.

Overall, these data suggest that the opiate antagonists—naloxone and naltrexone—are capable of inducing significant dose-dependent decreases in many of the symptoms associated with autism—including hyperactivity, stereotypy, and SIB—while, in some cases, enhancing the expression of appropriate social behavior. Clearly, additional studies are needed with more subjects, chronic administration of

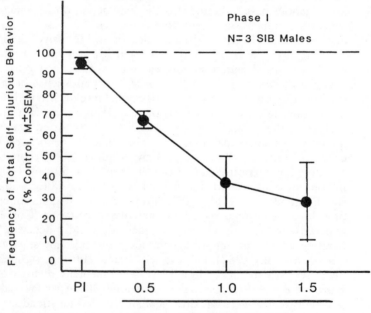

Figure 6-5. Mean frequency of total self-injurious behavior (SIB) for three male subjects after administration of placebo (PI) or naltrexone (.5, 1.0, and 1.5 mg/kg). Each test period was 5 minutes in duration. Types of SIBs included head and facial hits, facial gouging, self-biting, and other SIB responses, such as hand-to-leg hits and chin-to-shoulder hits (Herman et al. 1987; reprinted with permission from *Annals of Neurology* 22:550–552, 1987).

drugs, and double-blind designs to assess more carefully the effects of opiate antagonists on autism and SIB.

PROOPIOMELANOCORTIN-SEROTONIN MODEL FOR AUTISM

My group has postulated a novel biochemical model for autism that may offer an explanation of the link between abnormalities in POMC peptides and 5-HT in autism (Chamberlain and Herman 1990; Herman et al. 1986, 1988a). According to this model, the biological basis of autism may involve a hypersecretion of pineal melatonin, which results in a cascade of biochemical effects, including a corresponding hyposecretion of pituitary POMC peptides (Herman et al. 1986, 1987; Weizman et al. 1984, 1988), a hypersecretion of hypothalamic opioid peptides (Gillberg et al. 1985; Ross et al. 1987), and a hypersecretion of hypothalamic 5-HT (for blood studies, see Anderson et al. 1987; Campbell et al. 1975; Hanley et al. 1977; Ritvo et al. 1970; Schain and Freedman 1961; Takahashi et al. 1976; Young et al. 1982; Yuwiler et al. 1971; for fenfluramine studies, see August et al. 1987; Campbell et al. 1986a, 1986b; Ritvo et al. 1983, 1984, 1986; but see Campbell et al. 1987a, 1987b). Hypersecretion of pineal melatonin should produce a hypersecretion of 5-HT in the hypothalamus and blood (Anton-Tay et al. 1968). In addition, hypersecretion of melatonin would be expected to inhibit the release of corticotropin-releasing factor (Jones et al. 1976), which, in turn, should lead to decreased release of pituitary β-E and ACTH (Vale et al. 1981). This, in turn, should lead to decreased plasma concentrations of β-E, ACTH, and cortisol (Herman et al. 1986, 1988a; Weizman et al. 1984, 1988). In autism, a genetically determined hypersecretion of hypothalamic β-E (Ross et al. 1987) may further contribute to an inhibition of pituitary β-E because of negative-feedback inhibition between the hypothalamus and pituitary in the regulation of β-E. This model offers an explanation of the absence of a POMC stimulatory response to naltrexone in a majority of autistic individuals (Herman et al. 1988a, 1988b). In most autistic individuals, opioid receptor blockade by naltrexone may not signal the release for more opioids from the pituitary, since this system may be under continuous suppression by the negative-feedback inhibitory effects of hypersecreting hypothalamic opioid neurons. It is not surprising that only some autistic individuals show this POMC-naltrexone effect, since there is abundant evidence that autism represents a group of syndromes reflecting multiple biological etiologies.

Much additional research will be needed to determine the relationship between POMC peptides and 5-HT in autism; however, initial preclinical and clinical biochemical and pharmacological studies reviewed in this chapter have already started to provide the basis for a novel biochemical model for autism. Additional double-blind, controlled trials designed to determine the effects of naltrexone and fenfluramine in autism are needed, along with further biochemical studies designed to measure POMC peptides and 5-HT in blood, CSF, and the brain. With this two-pronged approach, perhaps at least a component of the etiology and treatment of this fascinating but perplexing disorder will be realized soon.

ACKNOWLEDGMENTS

I am grateful to Irene Chatoor, M.D., and James Egan, M.D., of Children's National Medical Center (CHNMC) for their astute and invaluable psychiatric diagnoses of the autistic and self-injurious subjects described in this report. Ann Arthur-Smith, B.S., provided expert technical assistance in the radioimmunoassays and the collection of some of the behavioral data. I am especially appreciative of the numerous students and research assistants who contributed to the collection of behavioral data in this report, including K. Appelgate, M.D., A. Werner, B.A., and J. Hartzler, B.A. Expert and scholarly assistance in the compilation of references in this report and unpublished manuscripts listed below was provided by Shirley S. Knobloch, R.N., M.L.S., and Deborah D. Gilbert, M.L.S., of Learning Resources of CHNMC. Ronald S. Chamberlain is the originator of the idea that a hypersecretion of pineal melatonin may be the originating biochemical dysregulation in SIB and autism. Our dreams for hope go to the children we treat and to the parents.

This chapter is based in part on preexisting unpublished text including the following: "The Effects of Naltrexone on Self-mutilation Behaviors and Autism in Children" by B.H. Herman et al. (CHNMC Institutional Review Board Research Protocol, March 26, 1984); "The Role of Opioids in Autism" by B.H. Herman et al. (NIH proposal, October 1, 1984); "The Role of Opioids in Autism and Self-injurious Behavior in Children" by B.H. Herman et al. (Stallone Fund for Autism Research, July 27, 1986); "Opioids in Self-injurious Behavior in Retarded Children" by B.H. Herman et al. (NICHD proposal, September 29, 1986); "The Role of Opioids in Autism" by B.H. Herman et al. (March of Dimes proposal, September 1, 1988); "Role of Opioids in Autistic Mentally Retarded Children" by B.H. Herman et al. (NICHD proposal, September 29, 1988); "Evaluation of Naltrexone in Autistic Children" by B.H. Herman et al. (FDA proposal, April 13, 1989); and "A Review of the Evidence Suggesting a Relationship Between Brain Proopiomelanocortin Peptides and

Serotonin in Autism" by B.H. Herman and R.S. Chamberlain (unpublished data, 1989).

This work was supported in part by Food and Drug Administration Orphan Drug Grant, NICH Grant HD23330-03, March of Dimes Birth Defects Social and Behavioral Sciences Research Grant 12-235, DuPont Pharmaceutical Grant, the Stallone Fund for Autism Research, the Board of Lady Visitors of the Children's National Medical Center, and the Adrianna Foundation (to B.H.H.).

REFERENCES

Adams SE: Naloxone reversal of analgesia produced by brain stimulation in the human. Pain 2:161–166, 1976

Akerly MS: The near-normal autistic adolescent. J Autism Childhood Schiz 4:347–356, 1974

Akil H, Watson SJ, Young E, et al: Endogenous opioids: biology and function. Ann Rev Neurosci 7:223–255, 1984

Aman MG, White AJ, Vaithianathan C, et al: Preliminary study of imipramine in profoundly retarded residents. Journal of Autism and Developmental Disorders 16:263–273, 1985

American Psychiatric Association: Diagnostic and Statistical Manual of Mental Disorders, 3rd Edition, Revised. Washington, DC, American Psychiatric Association, 1987

Anderson GM, Freedman DX, Cohen DJ, et al: Whole blood serotonin in autistics and normal subjects. J Child Psychol Psychiatry 28:885–900, 1987

Anderson LT, Campbell M, Grega DM, et al: Haloperidol in the treatment of infantile autism: effects on learning and behavioral symptoms. Am J Psychiatry 141:1195–1202, 1984

Anton-Tay F, Chou C, Anton S, et al: Brain serotonin concentration: elevation following intraperitoneal administration of melatonin. Science 162:277–278, 1968

August GJ, Raz N, Beard T: Fenfluramine response in high and low functioning autistic children. J Am Acad Child Adol Psychiatry 26:342–346, 1987

Barrett PR, Feinstein C, Hole WT: Effects of naloxone and naltrexone on self-injury: a double blind, placebo controlled analysis. Am J Ment Retard 93:644–651, 1989

Beckwith BE, Couk DI, Schumacher K: Failure of naloxone to reduce self-injurious behavior in two developmentally disabled females. Appl Res Ment Retard 7:183–188, 1986

Bell SM, Ainsworth MDS: Infant crying and maternal responsiveness. Child Dev 43:1171–1190, 1972

Belluzzi JD, Stein L: Enkephalin may mediate euphoria and drive-reduction reward. Nature 266:556–558, 1977

Bernstein GA, Hughes JR, Mitchell JE: Effects of narcotic antagonists on self-injurious behavior: a single case study. J Am Acad Child Adol Psychiatry 26:886–889, 1987

Blankstein J, Reyes FI, Winter JSD: Effects of naloxone on prolactin and cortisol in normal women. Proc Soc Exp Biol Med 164:363–365, 1980

Bortz WM II, Angwin P, Mefford IN: Catecholamines, dopamine and endorphin levels during extreme exercise. N Engl J Med 8:466–467, 1981

Bowlby J: Attachment and Loss, Vol 1. New York, Basic Books, 1969, p 256

Campbell M: Annotation: fenfluramine treatment of autism. J Child Psychol Psychiatry 29:1–10, 1988

Campbell M, Spencer EK: Psychopharmacology in child and adolescent psychiatry: a review of the past five years. J Am Acad Child Adol Psychiatry 27:269–279, 1988

Campbell M, Friedman E, Green WH: Blood serotonin in schizophrenic children: a preliminary study. Int Pharmacopsychiatry 10:213–221, 1975

Campbell M, Cohen IL, Anderson LT: Pharmacotherapy for autistic children: a summary of research. Can J Psychiatry 26:265–273, 1981

Campbell M, Deutch SL, Perry R, et al: Short-term efficacy and safety of fenfluramine in hospitalized preschoolage autistic children: an open study. Psychopharmacol Bull 22:141–147, 1986a

Campbell M, Perry R, Polonsky B: Brief report: an open study of fenfluramine in hospitalized young autistic children. J Autism Dev Disord 46:495–506, 1986b

Campbell M, Perry R, Small AM, et al: Overview of drug treatment in autism, in Neurobiological Issues in Autism. Edited by Schopler E, Mesibov GB. New York, Plenum Press, 1987a, pp 341–356

Campbell M, Small A, Palij M, et al: The efficacy and safety of fenfluramine in autistic children: preliminary analysis of a double-blind study. Psychopharmacol Bull 23:123–137, 1987b

Campbell M, Adams P, Small AM, et al: Naltrexone in infantile autism. Psychopharmacol Bull 24:135–139, 1988a

Campbell M, Adams P, Small A, et al: Efficacy and safety of fenfluramine in autistic children. J Am Acad Child Adol Psychiatry 4:434–439, 1988b

Campbell M, Overall JE, Small AM, et al: Naltrexone in autistic children: an acute open dose range tolerance trial. J Am Acad Child Adol Psychiatry 28:200–206, 1989

Carroll MN, Lim RKS: Observations on the neuropharmacology of morphine and morphine-like analgesia. Arch Int Pharmacodyn 125:383–403, 1960

Cataldo MF, Harris J: The biological basis for self-injury in the mentally retarded. Analysis and Intervention in Developmental Disabilities 2:21–39, 1982

Chamberlain RS, Herman BH: A novel biochemical model linking dysfunctions in brain melatonin, proopiomelanocortin peptides and serotonin in autism. Biol Psychiatry 28:773–793, 1990

Cohen C, Caparulo BK, Shaywitz BA, et al: Dopamine and serotonin metabolism in neuropsychiatrically disturbed children, CSF homovanillic acid and 5-hydroxyindoleacetic acid. Arch Gen Psychiatry 34:545–556, 1977

Coleman M, Gillberg C: The Biology of Autistic Syndromes. New York, Prager, 1985, p 25

Cox BM: Endogenous opioid peptides: a guide to structures and terminology. Life Sciences 31:1645–1658, 1982

Davidson PW, Kleene BM, Carroll M, et al: Effects of naloxone on self-injurious behavior: a case study. Appl Res Ment Retard 4:1–4, 1983

Delitala G, Devilla L, Aratal L: Opiate receptors and anterior pituitary hormone secretion in man: effect of naloxone infusion. Acta Endocrinol 97:150–156, 1981

Deutsch SI: Rationale for administration of opiate antagonists in treating infantile autism. Am J Ment Defic 90:631–635, 1986

Du Verglas G, Banks SR, Guyer KE: Clinical effects of fenfluramine on children with autism: a review of the research. J Autism Dev Dis 18:297–308, 1988

Freeman BJ, Ritvo ER, Guthrie D, et al: The Behavior Observation Scale for autism: initial methodology, data analysis and preliminary findings on 89 children. J Am Acad Child Psychiatry 17:576–583, 1978

Gillberg C, Svennerholm L, Hamilton-Helberg C: Childhood psychosis and monoamine metabolites in spinal fluid. Journal of Autism and Developmental Disorders 13:383–396, 1983

Gillberg C, Terenius I, Lunnerholm G: Endorphin activity in childhood psychosis. Arch Gen Psychiatry 42:780–783, 1985

Gispen-DeWied CC, Westenberg HG, Thijssen JH, et al: The dexamethasone and cortisol suppression test in depression: β-endorphin as a useful marker. Psychoneuroendocrinology 12:355–356, 1987

Goldstein A: Biology and chemistry of the dynorphin peptides, in The Peptides, Vol 6. Edited by Udenfriend S Jr, Meienhofer J. San Diego, CA, Academic, 1984, pp 95–145

Guillemin R, Vargo T, Rossier J, et al: β-endorphin and adrenocorticotropin are secreted concomitantly by the pituitary gland. Science 197:1367–1369, 1977

Hanley HG, Stahl SM, Freedman DX: Hyperserotonemia and amine metabolites in autistics and retarded children. Arch Gen Psychiatry 34:521–531, 1977

Harlow HF: The nature of love. Am Psychol 13:673–685, 1958

Herman BH: A possible role of proopiomelanocortin peptides in self-injurious behavior. Prog Neuro-Psychopharmacol Biol Psychiatry 14 (suppl):109–139, 1990

Herman BH, Goldstein A: Cataleptic effects of dynorphin-(1-13) in rats made tolerant to a mu opiate receptor agonist. Neuropeptides 2:13–22, 1981

Herman BH, Panksepp J: Effects of morphine and naloxone on social attachment in infant guinea pigs. Pharmacol Biochem Behav 9:213–220, 1978

Herman BH, Panksepp J: Ascending endorphin inhibition of distress vocalization. Science 221:1060–1062, 1981

Herman BH, Leslie F, Goldstein A: Behavioral effects and in vivo degradation of intraventricularly administered dynorphin-(1-13) and (D-Alaz) dynorphin-(1-11) in rats. Life Sci 27:883–892, 1980

Herman BH, Hammock MK, Egan J, et al: Naltrexone induces dose dependent decreases in self-injurious behavior. Soc Neurosci Abstr 11:468, 1985

Herman BH, Hammock MK, Arthur-Smith A: Role of opioid peptides in autism: effects of acute administration of naltrexone. Soc Neurosci Abstr 12:1172, 1986

Herman BH, Hammock MK, Arthur-Smith A, et al: Naltrexone decreases self-injurious behavior in children. Ann Neurol 22:550–552, 1987

Herman BH, Arthur-Smith A, Verebey K, et al: Effects of acute administration of naltrexone on plasma concentrations of naltrexone, 6-B-naltrexol, β-endorphin and cortisol in children. Soc Neurosci Abstr 14:465, 1988a

Herman BH, Arthur-Smith A, Hammock MK, et al: Ontogeny of β-endorphin and cortisol in the plasma of children and adolescents. J Clin Endocrinol Metab 67:186–190, 1988b

Herman BH, Hammock MK, Arthur-Smith A, et al: Effects of acute administration of naltrexone on cardiovascular function, body temperature, body weight and serum concentrations of liver enzymes in autistic children. Dev Pharmacol Ther 12:118–127, 1989a

Herman BH, Hammock MK, Egan J, et al: A role of opioid peptides in self-injurious behavior: dissociation from autonomic nervous system functioning. Dev Pharmacol Ther 12:81–89, 1989b

Holaday JW, Faden AI: Naltrexone reversal of endotoxin hypotension suggests role of endorphins in shock. Nature 275:450–451, 1978

Hollister LE, Johnson K, Boukhabza D, et al: Aversive effects of naltrexone in subjects not dependent on opiates. Drug Alcohol Depend 8:37–41, 1981

Hoshino Y, Ohno Y, Murata S: Dexamethasone suppression test in autistic children. Folia Psychiatr Neurol Japan 38:445–449, 1984

Hoshino Y, Yokoyama F, Watanabe M, et al: The diurnal variation and response to dexamethasone suppression test of saliva cortisol level in autistic children. Japan J Psychiatry Neurol 41:227–235, 1987

Houghton RA, Swan RW, Li CH: β-Endorphin: stability, clearance behavior, and entry into the central nervous system after intravenous injection of the tritiated peptide in rats and rabbits. Proc Natl Acad Sci USA 77:4588, 1980

Jensen JG, Realmuto GM, Garfinkle BD: The dexamethasone suppression test in infantile autism. J Amer Acad Child Psychiatry 24:263–265, 1985

Jones MT, Hillhouse E, Burden J: Effect of various putative neurotransmitters on the secretion of corticotrophin releasing hormone from the rat hypothalamus in vitro: a model of the neurotransmitters involved. Endocrinology 69:1–10, 1976

Judd LL, Janowsky L, Zettner DS, et al: Effects of naloxone-HCl on cortisol levels in patients with affective disorder and normal controls. Psychiatry Res 4:277–283, 1981

Kalat JW: Speculations on similarities between autism and opiate addiction (letter). J Autism Childhood Schiz 8:477–479, 1978

Kalin NH, Shelton SE: Defensive behaviors in infant rhesus monkeys: environmental cues and neurochemical regulation. Science 243:1718–1721, 1989

Kanner L: Autistic disturbance of affective content. Nerv Child 2:217–250, 1943

Kars H, Broekema W, Glaudemans-Van Gelderen I, et al: Naltrexone attenuates self-injurious behavior in mentally retarded subjects. Biol Psychiatry 27:741–746, 1990

Khachaturian H, Lewis ME, Tsou K, et al: β-Endorphin, alpha-MSH, ACTH, and related peptides, in Handbook of Chemical Neuroanatomy, Vol 4. Edited by Bjorkland A, Hokfelt T. New York, Elsevier, 1985, pp 216–272

Kosten TR, Kreek MJ, Ragunath J, et al: A preliminary study of beta endorphin during chronic naltrexone maintenance treatment in ex-opiate addicts. Life Sciences 39:55–59, 1986

Leboyer M, Bouvard MP, Dugas M: Effects of naltrexone on infantile autism. Lancet 1:715, 1988

Lee MC, Wagner HN, Tanada S, et al: Duration of occupancy of opiate receptors by naltrexone. J Nucl Med 29:1207–1211, 1988

Lundberg JM, Hokfelt T: Coexistence of peptides and classical neurotransmitters. Trends Neurosci 6:325–332, 1983

Mansour A, Khachaturian H, Lewis ME, et al: Anatomy of CNS opioid receptors. Trends Neurosci 11:308–314, 1988

Martin WR, Jasinski DR, Mansky PA: Naltrexone, an antagonist for the treatment of heroin dependence. Arch Gen Psychiatry 28:784–791, 1973

Mendelson JH, Ellingboe J, Keuhnle JC, et al: Effects of naltrexone on mood and neuroendocrine function in normal adult males. Psychoneuroendocrinology 3:231–236, 1979

Mendelson JH, Mello NK, Cristofaro P, et al: Use of naltrexone as a provacative test for hypothalamic-pituitary hormone function. Pharmacol Biochem Behav 24:309–313, 1986

Mitchell JE, Morley JE, Levine AS, et al: High-dose naltrexone therapy and dietary counseling for obesity. Biol Psychiatry 22:35–42, 1987

Morley JE, Baranetsky NG, Wingert TD, et al: Endocrine effects of naloxone induced opiate receptor blockade. J Clin Endocrinol Metab 50:251–257, 1980

O'Donohue TL, Dorsa DM: The opiomelanotropinergic neuronal and endocrine systems. Peptides 3:353–395, 1982

Panksepp J: A neurochemical theory of autism. Trends Neurosci 2:174–177, 1979

Panksepp J, DeEskinazi FG: Opiates and homing. J Comp Physiol Psychol 94:650–663, 1980

Panksepp J, Sahley TL: Possible brain opioid involvement in disrupted social intent and language development of autism, in Neurobiological Issues in Autism. Edited by Schopler E, Mesibov GB. New York, Plenum, 1987, pp 357–372

Panksepp J, Herman BH, Conner R, et al: The biology of social attachments: opiates alleviate separation distress. Biol Psychiatry 5:617–618, 1978a

Panksepp J, Herman BH, Vilberg T: An opiate excess model of childhood autism. Soc Neurosci Abstr 3:500, 1978b

Panksepp J, Vilberg T, Bean NB, et al: Reduction of distress vocalization in chicks by opiate-like peptides. Brain Res Bull 3:663–667, 1978c

Panksepp J, Meeker R, Bean NJ: The neurochemical control of crying. Pharmacol Biochem Behav 12:437–443, 1980a

Panksepp J, Herman BH, Vilberg T, et al: Endogenous opioids and social behavior. Neurosci Biobehav Rev 4:473–487, 1980b

Pfohl DN, Allen JI, Atkinson RL, et al: Naltrexone hydrochloride (Trexan): a review of serum transaminase elevations at high dosage. Natl Inst Drug Abuse Res Monogr Ser 67:66–72, 1986

Pomara N, Stanley M, Rhiew HB, et al: Loss of the cortisol response to naltrexone in Alzheimer's disease. Biol Psychiatry 23:726–733, 1988

Ratey J, Mikkelsen E, Smith GB, et al: Betablockers in the severely and profoundly mentally retarded. J Clin Psychopharmacol 6:103–107, 1986

Ratey JJ, Mikkelsen E, Sorgi P, et al: Autism: the treatment of aggressive behaviors. J Clin Psychopharmacol 7:35–41, 1987

Richardson JS, Zaleski NA: Naloxone and self-mutilation. Biol Psychiatry 18:99–101, 1983

Ritvo ER, Yuwiler A, Geller E, et al: Increased blood serotonin and platelets in early infantile autism. Arch Gen Psychiatry 23:556–572, 1970

Ritvo ER, Freeman BJ, Geller E, et al: Effects of fenfluramine on 14 outpatients with the syndrome of autism. Am J Psychiatry 142:74–77, 1983

Ritvo ER, Freeman BJ, Yuwiler A, et al: Study of fenfluramine in outpatients with the syndrome of autism. J Pediatr 105:823–828, 1984

Ritvo ER, Freeman BJ, Yuwiler A, et al: Fenfluramine treatment of autism: UCLA collaborative study of 81 patients at nine medical centers. Psychopharmacol Bull 22:133–140, 1986

Ross DL, Klykylo WM, Hitzeman R: Reduction of elevated CSF beta-endorphin by fenfluramine in infantile autism. Pediatr Neurol 3:83–86, 1987

Rossier J, French ED, Rivier C, et al: Foot shock-induced stress increases β-endorphin levels in blood but not in brain. Nature 270:618–620, 1977

Sandman CA: β-Endorphin disregulation in autistic and self-injurious behavior: a neurodevelopmental hypothesis. Synapse 2:193–199, 1988

Sandman CA, Datta PC, Barron J, et al: Naloxone attenutates self-abusive behavior in developmentally disabled clients. Appl Res Ment Retard 4:5–11, 1983

Sandman CA, Barron JL, Crinella FM, et al: Influence of naloxone on brain and behavior of a self-injurious woman. Biol Psychiatry 22:899–906, 1987

Sandyk R: Naloxone abolished self-injuring in a mentally retarded child. Ann Neurol 17:520, 1985

Schain RJ, Freedman D: Studies on 5-hydroxyindol metabolism in autistic and other mentally retarded children. J Pediatr 58:315–320, 1961

Schlachter LB, Wardlaw SL, Tindall GT, et al: Persistence of β-endorphin in human cerebrospinal fluid after hypophysectomy. J Clin Endocrinol Metab 57:221–224, 1983

Sigman M, Mundy P: Social attachments in autistic children. J Am Acad Child Adol Psychiatry 28:74–81, 1989

Singh NN, Millichamp CJ: Pharmacological treatment of self-injurious behavior in mentally retarded persons. Journal of Autism and Developmental Disorders 15:257–267, 1985

Snyder SH: Drug and neurotransmitter receptors in the brain. Science 224:22–31, 1984

Szymanski L, Kedesdy J, Sulkes S, et al: Naltrexone in treatment of self-injurious behavior: a clinical study. Res Dev Dis 8:179–190, 1987

Takahashi S, Kanai H, Miyamoto Y: Reassessment of elevated serotonin levels in blood platelets in early infantile autism. J Autism Childhood Schiz 6:317–326, 1976

Todd RD, Ciaranello RD: Demonstration of inter- and intra-species difference in serotonin binding sites by antibodies from autistic children. Arch Gen Psychiatry 39:174–180, 1985

Vale W, Spiess J, Rivier C, et al: Characterization of 41-residue ovine hypothalamic peptide that stimulates secretion of corticotropin and β-endorphin. Science 213:1394–1397, 1981

Verebey K, Mule SJ: Naltrexone and β-naltrexol plasma levels in schizophrenic patients after large oral doses of naltrexone. Res Comm Psychol Psychiatr Behav 4:311–317, 1979

Verebey K, Volavka J, Mule SJ, et al: Naltrexone: disposition, metabolism, and effects after acute and chronic dosing. Clin Pharmacol Ther 20:315–328, 1976

Watson SJ, Barchas JD, Li CH: Beta-lipotropin: localization in cells and axons in rat brain by immunocytochemistry. Proc Natl Acad Sci USA 74:5155–5158, 1977

Weizman R, Weizman A, Tyano S, et al: Humoral-endorphin blood levels in autistic schizophrenic and healthy subjects. Psychopharmacology 82:368–370, 1984

Weizman R, Gil-Ad I, Dick J, et al: Low plasma immunoreaction β-endorphin levels in autistics. J Am Acad Child Adol Psychiatry 27:430–433, 1988

Young JG, Kavanagh ME, Anderson GM, et al: Clinical neurochemistry of autism and other disorders. J Autism Dev Disord 12:147–165, 1982

Yuwiler A, Freedman DX: Neurotransmitter research in autism, in Neurobiological Issues in Autism. Edited by Schopler E, Mesibov GB. New York, Plenum, 1987, pp 263–284

Yuwiler A, Ritvo ER, Bald D, et al: Examination of circadian rhythmicity of blood serotonin and platelets in autistic and non-autistic children. J Autism Childhood Schiz 1:421–435, 1971

Yuwiler A, Ritvo ER, Geller E, et al: Uptake and efflux of serotonin from platelets of autistic and non-autistic children. J Autism Childhood Schiz 8:83–98, 1975

Zelnik N, Herman BHH, Hammock MK: Role of opioid peptides in self-injurious behavior. Soc Neurosci Abstr 12:412, 1986

Chapter 7

Amantadine: Profile of Use in the Developmentally Disabled

Mark Chandler, M.D., L. Jarrett Barnhill, M.D., and C. Thomas Gualtieri, M.D.

Amantadine (1-adamantanamine or 1-aminotricyclo-$[3.3.1.1^{3,7}]$ - decane) hydrochloride is a water-soluble salt that apparently penetrates all cell membranes, including those of the central nervous system. There is a growing body of information on amantadine treatment for neuropsychiatric patients. The most firmly established uses are the prevention of influenza A in healthy young adults and the treatment of Parkinson's disease. Amantadine is among the accepted approaches for management of several side effects to neuroleptic drugs. Mentally retarded people suffer from numerous difficult-to-manage behaviors, including agitation and severe disorganization. Stimulant medications have been used to treat patients with developmental disabilities, but there is considerable controversy as to their efficacy. Certain characteristics of amantadine, notably the direct dopaminergic action, might permit beneficial action where stimulants do not. We present a series of case reports of patients with developmental disabilities and attempt to clarify some of the features that might identify patients with amantadine-responsive conditions.

Early History

The preparation of amantadine derivatives was extensively explored by Stetter (1954). Of the many adamantine derivatives, only amantadine hydrochloride has been widely studied for human use. The antiviral action was explored during the 1960s and early 1970s (Galbraith et al. 1970). The efficacy of amantadine in Parkinson's disease was discovered serendipitously in 1968 when a 58-year-old woman with moderately severe Parkinson's disease was taking amantadine to prevent the flu. She experienced a remarkable remission in her symptoms of rigidity, tremor, and akinesia. These problems recurred promptly after stopping the drug. Schwab et al. (1969) did preliminary testing in 10 patients. Seven of these patients showed marked reduction in akinesia, lessening of tremor, and some improvement in rigidity, with no side effects reported.

Mechanism of Action

It is generally accepted that amantadine acts presynaptically to enhance dopamine (DA) release or inhibit DA reuptake without any direct effect on DA receptors (Gianutsos et al. 1985). On the other hand, there is additional information to suggest a direct, postsynaptic effect, perhaps to increase the density of postsynaptic DA receptors (Gianutsos et al. 1985) or to alter the conformation of the DA receptor (Allen 1983). Stromberg and Svensson (1970) noted a specific inhibitory effect of amantadine on cortical and striatal neurons when applied microiontophoretically. In various animal models, amantadine appears to behave as a competitive blocker of the receptor effects of apomorphine and amphetamine (Allen 1983). There is evidence that presynaptic antagonism of indirect-acting stimulants occurs with amantadine (Menon et al. 1973). In some animal models, amantadine abolishes the hyperactivity (Prepas et al. 1985) and high-intensity stereotyped behavior (Cox and Tha 1973) induced by d-amphetamine. The mechanism of action of amantadine in parkinsonism is reviewed by Bailey and Stone (1975).

It would seem, therefore, that the dopaminergic effects of the drug represent a combination of direct (postsynaptic) and indirect (presynaptic) influences. The relative weighting of such effects for the various dopamine agonists would account, then, for their overlapping but not necessarily identical clinical profiles (Schneiden and Cox 1976). Although there may be stimulatory effects on noradrenaline receptors (Papeschi 1974), the most meaningful influence on the behavior appears to be via dopaminergic systems (Allen 1983).

The mechanism of the antiviral action is thought to be interference with the penetration of the host cell by the virus (Davies et al. 1964). The phagocytosis of viral particles may be prevented, ionic changes at the cell membrane may be caused, or viral receptor areas on cell membranes may be blocked with amantadine use (Dales and Choppin 1962; Papeschi 1974). It is not clear that any of these effects contribute to neurotherapeutic effects.

RATIONALE FOR USE IN THE DEVELOPMENTALLY DISABLED

Agitation, inattention, irritability, screaming, self-injury, and aggressive behavior are, unfortunately, common referral problems to a neuropsychiatry clinic in a mental retardation center. In such cases, there is a limited number of treatment options available. In instances when these symptoms are mild, they are dealt with behaviorally. Medication alternatives are usually the β-blockers, the psychotropic anticonvulsants, and lithium. Other alternatives are stimulant medications, naltrexone, clonidine, and L-tryptophan. Clopenthixol decanoate has recently been suggested for management of aggressive mentally disabled patients (Mlele et al. 1986). Neuroleptic medications may be prescribed, but in light of their many serious problems— such as neuroleptic malignant syndrome and tardive dyskinesia— other alternatives are sought. Each of the existing treatment options has problems in some patients. β-Blockers may cause hypotension, necessitating discontinuation of the medication. Anticonvulsants may, in some instances, cause liver damage or severe skin reactions. Lithium may cause hypothyroidism or cardiac arrhythmia in some people.

Presynaptic DA agonists, such as methylphenidate and dextroamphetamine, have been reported to be of some use for behavioral disorders of mild to moderately mentally retarded people (Alexandris and Lundell 1968; Blacklidge and Ekblad 1971; Varley and Trupin 1982); however, most studies suggest stimulant medications are not helpful in mentally retarded people, particularly the severe and profoundly retarded (Aman and Singh 1982; Bell and Zubek 1961; Davis et al. 1969).

Most studies of stimulant medications used in the clinical management of autistic children have been negative (Campbell 1975, 1976). Dextroamphetamine caused a worsening of stereotypes in these children (Aman 1982; Campbell 1975).

All of the effort invested in stimulant research is probably due to evidence that frontal dopamine systems are involved in disorders of memory, impulse control, and planning. Malfunctioning dopamine systems have been implicated in the etiology of aggressive behavior (Maeda et al. 1975; Pradham 1975). A fundamental piece of information is that the destruction of dopaminergic pathways with 6-hydroxydopamine produced increased hyperactivity, irritability, and aggression in low doses, whereas higher doses produced tremor, rigidity, and convulsions in cats (Beleslin et al. 1981). Animal work suggests that DA agonists may produce functional recovery from septal lesions that effect hypothalamic defensive attack (Maeda et al. 1987) and other behaviors (Lungberg and Ungerstedt 1976; Marotta et al. 1977; Marshall and Gotthelf 1979; Marshall and Ungerstedt 1976).

Mental retardation may involve dysfunction of a host of monoamine neurotransmitter systems that project to the cortex and striatum and that mediate fundamental aspects of cortical arousal.

Monoamine central nervous system transmission deficiencies are thought to occur in some mentally retarded patients. Patients with cerebral palsy with physical evidence of subcortical injury are a group of particular interest. We began clinical trials with amantadine in developmentally disabled patients with evidence of subcortical injury, severe inattention, and irritability or abulia unresponsive to other treatments.

Amantadine is a compound worth considering for patients with severe agitation, particularly if the agitation is unresponsive to other interventions or side effects have ended an earlier drug trial. The dose range is narrow (adults, 100–400 mg per day; children, 4.4–8.8 mg/kg per day), the onset of therapeutic action is relatively quick (4 days at each dose increment), the side-effect profile is favorable, monitoring is a simple task, and there are not many troublesome drug interactions to worry about (Bean 1986). It is a reasonable option to add to a neuroleptic medicine to permit tapering of the DA blocker. Amantadine is not a sedating drug, an important consideration in patients with cognitive dysfunction. If behavior toxicity develops on amantadine, the effect is readily reversible when the drug is withdrawn. There is some experience in other difficult-to-treat populations on which clinicians using amantadine can draw. We review the known uses of amantadine in detail to provide an experiential background for our clinical trials.

CLINICAL USE FOR NEUROPSYCHIATRIC PROBLEMS

Amantadine is becoming an increasingly popular drug among neurologists and other neuroscientists. The drug appears to have influences on cognition, motor performance, and social behavior. As this medication gains more use, more patients with severe behavioral disorders are discovered to benefit from treatment. What patients would do better with amantadine than with existing approaches? There have been clinical reports and small clinical studies to guide the use of amantadine for other neuropsychiatric conditions.

Those patients with Parkinson's disease who have symptoms of rigidity and akinesia are most likely to respond to amantadine (Harvey 1986). Among amantadine responders, there will often be a moderate decline in clinical efficacy during the first months of treatment (Schwab et al. 1972). The drug has stimulating properties, and amantadine-treated patients report that they feel more lively and alert when using the drug (Schwab et al. 1972). The major side effects of the drug are stimulant-like: irritability, agitation, disorganization, and psychosis. These four elements are reflected in the wider clinical profile of the drug.

As an anti-Parkinson's disease agent, it appears to exercise a more potent effect than the anticholinergic drugs, with fewer side effects (Harvey 1986). For example, anticholinergic drugs are known to impair memory performance, an important consideration in the treatment of elderly patients. Amantadine, compared with benzotropine, does not impair memory in healthy volunteers who are young (Van Putten et al. 1987) or elderly (McEvoy et al. 1987). It is as effective as the anticholinergics for the acute side effects of neuroleptic treatment, but it is free of any atropinelike side effects, so it may be preferable in many, if not most, clinical situations (Borison 1983; Fann and Lake 1976; Gelenberg 1978; Stenson et al. 1976).

In the treatment of neuroleptic-induced extrapyramidal disorders, amantadine is most effective for pseudo-Parkinson's disease, bradykinesia, abulia, rigidity, and akinesia and relatively less effective for dystonia and akathisia (Ananth et al. 1977; Borison 1983; Gelenberg and Mandell 1977; Kelley and Abuzzahab 1971). It is also used to treat tardive dyskinesia (Jankowsky 1973).

Amantadine has been shown to antagonize neuroleptic-induced prolactin elevation, indicating an effect on pituitary DA receptors, and may be a form of treatment for galactorrhea in patients who appear absolutely to need neuroleptic treatment (Siever 1981).

The activating properties of amantadine have led to trials for patients with "negative" symptoms of schizophrenia (withdrawal, abulia, and bradykinesia), and in this application the drug is about as useful as the other DA agonists (Angrist et al. 1980; Davidoff and Reifenstein 1939; Kornetsky 1976). It is occasionally effective in neuroleptic-induced catatonia (Gelenberg and Mandel 1977). It is found to be effective for the fatigue and depression that accompany multiple sclerosis (Murray 1985). Antagonism of ethanol-evoked responses by amantadine has been noted (Messiha 1978).

Amantadine appears to be a treatment for Jakob-Creutzfeldt disease, a slow viral disease, and has been tried in numerous other virus-related conditions, such as subacute sclerosing panencephalitis (Braham 1971).

Treatment with the more-potent agonist bromocriptine improved the level of arousal in a man with akinetic mutism (Ross and Stewart 1981), alleviated symptoms of neglect in two patients with right-hemisphere infarcts (Fleet et al. 1987), and was successful for neuroleptic malignant syndrome (Granato et al. 1983; Lazarus 1984; Simpson and David 1985).

Amantadine is effective for the treatment of one cerebral dysmaturation syndrome, nocturnal enuresis (Ambrosini and Fried 1984), but its effect in another, attention-deficit/hyperactivity, is equivocal (Mattes 1980). Amantadine has been used with some success for Tourette's syndrome (Borison 1983).

The use of DA agonists, their effect on cortical recovery, and their indications for patients with neurobehavioral sequelae of a brain injury have been discussed earlier (Evans and Gualtieri 1987; Gualtieri 1988). We have suggested that a mixed presynaptic and postsynaptic DA agonist, such as amantadine, may have particular utility in patients with extensive subcortical injury (Chandler et al. 1988). Our idea is that when the presynaptic neuron is severely damaged or dysfunctional, the effects of a presynaptic agonist cannot be sustained. We reported a marked reduction of agitation and assaultive behavior with amantadine in two patients with frontotemporal lesions after a closed head injury (Chandler et al. 1988). The extent of the improvement of these two young men, whose difficulties arose during the transitional stage of coma recovery, was surprising.

TOXICITY

The toxicity profile for amantadine is favorable, especially when it is compared with alternative treatments. As an antiviral agent, it has had wide use and little serious toxicity in children, elderly adults, and the mentally disabled (MMWR 1987; Reines and Gross 1988). A careful review of known side effects is essential for safe use of a medication in a novel population. Therefore, an exhaustive list of reported side effects is provided.

Behavioral toxicity has been the most important side effect, and it appears to have limited the use of amantadine in some patients who need it the most. Behavioral symptoms include insomnia, vivid dreams, anorexia, hallucinations, irritability, nervousness, agitation, disorganization, psychosis, hyperactivity, aggression, delirium, and depression (Borison 1979; Nestlebaum et al. 1986; Safta et al. 1976). The symptoms remit when the dose is lowered or the drug is discontinued (Harper and Knothe 1973; Mulser et al. 1975; Rizzo and Morselli 1972; Schwab et al. 1969).

Amantadine has been considered as a treatment for the neuropsychiatric problems associated with dementia. This makes sense, first, because the behavioral symptoms that occur in these conditions are sometimes similar to those we know improve in patients with Parkinson's disease and, second, because DA agonists are believed to enhance at least some aspects of cortical recovery from (or accommodation to) a neuropathic process (Gualtieri and Evans 1988; Feeney et al. 1982). The clinical work that has been done in this area, however, has not been enlightening. The results of clinical trials of amantadine and of memantine, a closely related derivative (Meldrum et al. 1986; Reiser et al. 1988), have not been encouraging. There have been reports of reduced agitation and improved alertness and function in demented patients treated with amantadine (Muller et al. 1979), but therapeutic effects have been compromised by the frequent occurrence of behavioral toxicity (Fleischhacker et al. 1986). The elderly may metabolize the drug differently or be more sensitive to toxic effects.

Schwab et al. (1969, 1972) described seizures as a high-dose side effect of amantadine, and we have observed the same association in clinical experience with head-injury patients. Anticonvulsant activity of memantine has been observed in animal models (Reiser et al. 1988). Dopamine agonists are usually associated with a higher seizure threshold, and there is one influential report that has claimed benefit for amantadine in the treatment of refractory epilepsy in childhood (Shields et al. 1985). Other dopamine agonists may have anticonvulsant properties (Livingston et al. 1973).

Amantadine has been used in the treatment of tardive dyskinesia (Allen 1982); however, abrupt discontinuation of amantadine in patients using neuroleptics may precipitate severe toxicity, including neuroleptic malignant syndrome (Hamburg et al. 1986). Amantadine interaction with dyazide may cause confusion and ataxia (Wilson and Rajput 1983). Amantadine overdose is associated with cardiac arrhythmia, for example, torsade de pointe (Sartori 1984). Interaction with phenelzine may cause severe hypertension. Neurotoxicity may be enhanced by simultaneous use of anticholinergic agents or antihistamines (Millet et al. 1982).

Livedo reticularis is a skin disorder characterized by a marbled mottled appearance with many causes. It was first noted in amantadine-treated patients with Parkinson's disease by Shealy et al. (1970). Livedo may be present in 60% of the healthy population older than 50 years (Vollum et al. 1971). After 6–8 weeks of amantadine treatment for Parkinson's disease, 90% developed livedo or existent livedo worsened. Livedo reticularis usually does not persist after amantadine withdrawal (Papeschi 1974).

Again, this is an exhaustive list of side effects. Any medication held to this degree of scrutiny will have instances of serious side effects. Nevertheless, amantadine has been safely used in a range of patients exceeding most other drugs. The side-effect profile compares favorably with alternatives, such as neuroleptic drugs that have a high incidence of debilitating consequences.

PHARMACOKINETICS

Amantadine is almost completely absorbed (the site not determined), and peak plasma concentrations occur 1–4 hours after ingestion (Aoki and Sitar 1985, 1988; Aoki et al. 1985; Montanari et al. 1975; Wu et al. 1982). Clearance is renal (Bleidner et al. 1965; Wu et al. 1982). Patients with kidney disease and decreased drug clearance are more prone to toxicity (Ing et al. 1979, 1980; Hordam et al. 1981; Postma and Van Tilburg 1975). Early reports suggested that humans did not metabolize amantadine (Bleiner et al. 1965); however the drug may be acetylated (Koppel and Tenczer 1985). Distribution is through all of the tissues of the body, including the central nervous system. Serum-level testing is available, but there is little known about therapeutic range.

THERAPEUTIC TRIALS

Our data are best viewed as case reports. That is, clinical trials of amantadine were instituted after a patient had done poorly on many other drugs and continued to exhibit extremely disruptive behavior. We carefully monitored target behaviors, side effects, and social functioning. Two case reports are presented.

Case Reports

One of our patients is an 11-year-old boy with mild mental retardation (full-scale IQ by WISC-R is 59), unknown etiology, articulation difficulties, stuttering, and fine and gross motor deficits. Chromosome testing for fragile X was negative. A recent magnetic resonance imaging scan of the head was normal, as was intensive video electroencephalogram (EEG) monitoring. His adaptive behavior is severely impaired by extreme hyperactivity and temper tantrums. Past medications for behavioral management included carbamazepine, valproic acid, Xanax, Mellaril, and Haldol. Behavior on each medication remained severely disruptive. A trial of amantadine was begun at 50 mg twice per day and gradually increased to 100 mg three times per day. The boy's parents reported a decrease of tantrums, improved attention, and improved ability to work with other children. He developed livedo reticularis 4 months into amantadine treatment. The drug was tapered for a 2-week period. Marked behavioral deterioration occurred with severe tantrums, and tremendous hyperactivity lasted 4 weeks after amantadine was discontinued. He was hospitalized, and amantadine was reinstituted after a dermatology consultation was obtained. The livedo reticularis cleared briefly but recurred 2 months after the drug was restarted. Behavior problems have decreased sufficiently so that he can live at home, but his parents still must make tremendous efforts to structure his time.

Another patient is a severely retarded 22-year-old blind male. The causes of his mental retardation and blindness are unknown. A routine EEG was normal. Behavior problems have included episodes of severe agitation and self-injurious behavior, particularly head banging and hand biting with tissue damage. Self-injurious behavior occurred 20–40 times per month before amantadine treatment and decreased 0–2 incidents per month for the next 6 months while the patient was taking the drug.

Although these are preliminary data, this case suggests that a direct-acting DA agonist may benefit some severely retarded patients. Because pharmacotherapy for behavior disorders in the severely retarded is a developing field, this is an interesting observation that must be followed by longer assessment and controlled studies.

The patients described in Table 7-1 have developmental disabilities with varying severity. They had persistent, severe behavioral disorders that failed to respond to behavioral and environmental intervention. Most had received several previous medication trials, although not all trials had been done under our care. The list in Table 7-1 includes all mentally retarded patients treated with amantadine seen through our consultation service, either in a clinic or at a residential mental retardation center. The observations from the clinical trials of amantadine are summarized in Table 7-2. Of the 28 individuals receiving amantadine, 10 had a positive response with no significant side effects, 11 had a partial response but the drug efficacy was limited by side effects, and 7 had no response or were worse with the drug. The side effects experienced by patients are summarized in Table 7-2.

Several of these patients had severe agitation, aggression, and hyperactivity. The response of these patients agrees with our experience with head-injured people, whose symptoms of agitation were reduced by amantadine. In contrast to the experience of Muller et al. (1979), we found that the occurrence of behavioral toxicity in patients with head injuries was quite low.

The response of agitation with amantadine is consistent with the hypothesis that subcortical dopaminergic neurotransmission is severely impaired in some mentally retarded patients, that direct stimulation of striatal and cortical DA neurons can lend a degree of higher regulatory support, and that it is possible to improve cognitive processing and alleviate confusion, disorganization, and dismay with amantadine treatment and thus reduce the occurrence of severe target behaviors, such as agitation and assaultiveness.

The treatment of organic agitation, however, does not reflect the

Table 7-1. Amantadine report

Name	Age (years)	Diagnosis/target behavior	Results	Response category
TC	12	Moderate MR; CP; ADHD Hearing deficit SZ disorder (grand mal)	Decreased aggression Increased compliance Developed skin rash; briefly later the rash resolved	R
JA	5	Congenital toxoplasma infection Chorioretinitis Low normal IQ SZ with left frontal focus Severe ADHD	Improved attention and hyperactivity No seizures witnessed to date Enuresis continues	R
JB	9	ADHD IQ in borderline range Specific language disorder	Greatly improved with less activity Aggression and tantrums decreased Rare upset stomach	R
ZW	17	Severe MR Autism Destructive and hyperactive	Mild change in aggressive behavior Improved attention and socialization Tried taper but behaviors worsened	R
TM		Severe MR Autism Hyperactive and aggressive Dysphoric	Last seen in our clinic 11/88 "Doing great" No side effects	R

CB	32	Severe MR Right hemiparesis second to CP SIB	Improved flexibility Weight loss of 20 pounds in 4 months No change in appetite	PR/SE
CQ	8	Autism Hyperactive; SIB; aggression Low average IQ Congenital hydrocephalus	Did well on amantadine until developed loss of appetite, insomnia, and irritability	PR/SE
BR	13	Moderate MR Yelling; aggression; ADHD SZ disorder with temporal focus Enuresis	Aggression and hyperactivity much improved Developed livedo reticularis Behavior deteriorated when discontinued amantadine, improved when amantadine restarted	PR/SE
MB	64	Moderate CP with left hemiparesis Possible tardive dyskinesia Right frontal, right caudate Infarcts by CT	Initially decreased rigidity More attentive and more cooperative Developed upset stomach	PR/SE
RW		Mild MR Staring spells Hyperactivity; mild SIB Possible SZ disorder	Decreased overactivity and noncompliance Slight increase in staring spells Fewer tantrums	PR/SE
NP	23	IQ in borderline range ADHD	100 mg twice per day; noted improved attention 100 mg three times per day; motivation and organization improved	R

continued

Table 7-1. Amantadine report (continued)

Name	Age (years)	Diagnosis/target behavior	Results	Response category
JB	9	Specific language disability Pervasive developmental delay Borderline intellectual functioning Hx psychogenic water drinking Multiple episodes of lipid pneumonia	Much improved; decrease in tantrums Better concentration; improved cooperation Improved social relatedness	R
RH		Asthma Mild MR Failure to thrive; encopresis Waxy flexibility; flat affect Cogwheeling; juvenile Parkinson's disease	More spontaneous; more fluid movements More energy and initiative	R
JM	11	Severe MR Autism Hyperactive and disorganized Aggression	Decreased aggression Less agitated on current dose, although both better than baseline	R
LP	37	Mild MR Abulia alternating with rages	Decreased rages; less anxious Appetite better	R
BD	8	Autism Mild MR ADHD Cystinuria	Improved school performance Virtually eliminated SIB Weight loss; decreased appetite	PR/SE

EH	13	Mild MR ADHD; tantrums Sudden mood swings Use of diapers and other regressive behaviors	Improved attention and cooperation Decreased aggression Mild stomach upset occasionally Stopped because of reports that TCA is better	PR/SE
BJ	6	Pervasive developmental delay Specific language disability ADHD Borderline intellectual function	Initial mild-to-moderate improvement but required residential setting Appetite loss at higher doses	PR/SE
GD		Severe MR Autism Intermittently explosive Agitated disorders	Initially did very well on lower dose but needed to gradually increase dose as irritability would reappear	PR/SE
JB		Autism Migraine headaches Abulia; bradykinesia Cogwheeling etiology unknown	Low doses (50 mg twice per day) associated with more energy and surprisingly fewer headaches Cogwheeling decreased Worse when amantadine decreased Appetite loss	PR/SE
TL		Moderate MR Williams syndrome Hyperactive and irritable	Initial mild response but MPH felt better	PR/SE
DA	14	Autism Severe MR Grand mal seizures	SIB worse; tearfulness worse; dysphoria	Worse

Table 7-1. Amantadine report (continued)

Name	Age (years)	Diagnosis/target behavior	Results	Response category
RA	7	Mild MR ADHD	Stopped when behavior worsened on low doses More restless and irritable	Worse
SW		Profound MR Autistic features	More agitation and irritability Tantrums increased	Worse
JK	57	Severe MR Hx of bacterial meningitis NMS, multiple episodes Episodic agitation and aggression	Bradykinesia improved but entered state that progressed to catatonia and NMS while on amantadine also did same on CBZ and LICO$_3$	NR
SP	25	Profound MR Hx epiglottis Left facial hematrophy Hyperactivity and agitation	Started by outside physician for flu prevention; stopped after little change No side effects	NR
EH	22	Moderate MR Episodes of severe agitation Public masturbation	Little change; less social withdrawal Combative behavior and irritability continued	NR
RL		Profound MR; autism Agitation; SIB Masturbation	Thorazine taper tried but severe with increased agitation	NR

Note. The response categories are positive responders (R), partial responders/side effects (PR/SE), no response (NR), and worse. CP, cerebral palsy; SZ, seizure; MPH, methylphenidate; CBZ, carbamazepine; LICO$_3$, lithium carbonate; CT, computerized tomography; TCA, tricyclic anticonvulsant; Hx, history; NMS, neuroleptic malignant syndrome.

cardinal indications for amantadine in Parkinson's disease, which are akinesia, abulia, rigidity, and low arousal. We have had the opportunity to test the efficacy of amantadine for mentally retarded people with neurobehavioral symptoms that fit this template.

Among the patients described in Table 7-1 was a group of mentally retarded people with predominant bradykinesia, abulia, or low arousal. The usual recommendation for such patients is a trial of stimulants or antidepressants. Amantadine was prescribed, in preference to those agents, because the patients were more severely impaired and the prescription of presynaptic agonists—stimulants and antidepressants—had been of little avail. The improvement of these negative symptoms was mild in contrast to the changes seen in agitated people. Perhaps high-threshold behaviors, such as aggression, are much more notable when removed. We observed some increased ability to socialize and participate in habilitation but no change that altered a patient's placement.

This is a small group of patients with several people showing a marked reduction in agitated, disruptive behavior. More patients showed side effects outweighing benefits. This is not unusual in difficult-to-treat populations with disorders that, in all likelihood, have multiple causes. A behavior response within a few days after starting use of a drug in a person whose behavior has been out of control despite many previous drug trials is a convincing clinical experience.

DISCUSSION

Dopamine agonists, particularly direct-acting dopaminergic agents such as amantadine, offer a different clinical profile than agents now routinely used for behavior disorders in the mentally retarded. The therapeutic profile of amantadine is expanded to include patient

Table 7-2. Observations from clinical trials of amantadine

n	Observation
28	Patients of various degrees of developmental disabilities
10	Positive response; no significant side effects
11	Partial response; treatment limited by side effects
7	No response or worse with drug

Note. Diagnosis, severity of developmental disability, sex, and age did not predict response. One patient with frontal seizure focus responded; a patient with a temporal lobe focus did not. Side effects included stomach upset (5 patients), loss of appetite (3), weight loss (2), insomnia (1), irritability (5), dysphoria (1), and livedo reticularis (1). These adverse reactions were not severe and cleared with discontinuation of medication.

groups not previously considered: mentally disabled individuals with symptoms of agitation and abulia. These preliminary observations are best viewed as case reports and require further development under controlled circumstances, but the proper design of controlled studies can only come after a period of clinical observation and the necessary accumulation of basic information about the drug, its likely indications, problems with treatment, and consequences of long-term treatment.

We have mentioned some of the practical advantages of amantadine treatment, but it is appropriate to list a few more at this point. First, amantadine is a "yes-no" drug; either it works or it does not. When it does work, the effects are usually dramatic. It is not simply a mild tranquilizer that "takes the edge off" a troublesome behavior pattern. If a patient is not substantially improved, there is no reason to continue use of the drug. Thus, there should be no difficulty in detecting the positive effects of treatment using more systematic measures than the clinical observations on which we have relied. Second, therapeutic effects often come quickly, within a matter of days, and dose increments of 50 mg to 100 mg per day can be made at weekly intervals to a maximum total daily dose of 400 mg per day, so it should not take long before the effects are apparent.

Third, toxicity is overt, not covert, as it is for such drugs as neuroleptics and phenytoin. The major side effects are behavioral toxicity, gastrointestinal side effects, and seizures. They are reversible when the drug is discontinued, and it may be discontinued over a week's time if that is necessary. One patient developed livedo reticularis after 3 months of using amantadine. The livedo cleared after 6 weeks of not using the drug, but the patient's behavior deteriorated to the point where institutionalization would have been required had the drug not been restarted.

Fourth, the drug is not sedating. It does not confer behavioral improvement at the expense of cognitive impairment. In fact, patients appear to be more alert and attentive in therapies of various sort.

Fifth, the drug may improve motor performance by reducing rigidity, even in patients who have had this symptom for years. This effect makes amantadine particularly interesting in the clinical care of cerebral palsy patients.

Sixth, we have not seen significant worsening of stereotypes or self-stimulatory behavior. This issue will demand careful testing, because stereotypical behaviors can impair many habilitation efforts.

The design of a placebo-controlled, double-blind study of amantadine effects, with objective measures of behavioral and neuropsychological improvement, should not, then, be difficult. Such a study, however, should necessarily include a prolonged follow-up period for amantadine responders, since there is an occasional falloff in effect over months, as there is, on occasion, among patients with Parkinson's disease.

Our experience with amantadine is entirely anecdotal, so much more must be determined about the parameters of amantadine treatment. The extreme heterogeneity of our patient groups should serve as a caution for one theorizing from this data.

One is impelled, however, to theorize about amantadine effects in special patient populations by the arguments made in favor of a direct DA agonist in the treatment of patients with subcortical lesions. In certain classes of patients, it is reasonable to surmise that the presynaptic neuron is incapable of supporting the action of an indirect agonist, whereas the striatal or cortical neuron retains at least a limited capacity to respond to the agency of direct stimulation. This is an inference borrowed from the therapeutic physiology of Parkinson's disease, and its validity would not be proven even if the clinical observations contained herein were supported by controlled studies. After all, the precise nature of the dopaminergic action of amantadine is incompletely understood. But it represents, if not a testable hypothesis, at least a rationale for further investigation.

The psychopharmacological model for dopaminergic treatment is the use of stimulant drugs for hyperactivity. But there is an interesting aspect of stimulant treatment that is well established in developmental neuropsychiatry and that is germane to our reflections on amantadine and its therapeutic utility. Hyperactive children who are well endowed intellectually respond well to stimulants; as one descends the ladder of cognitive ability, however, the response is diminished. Mildly retarded children respond less well to stimulants, moderately retarded children respond only on rare occasions, and severely retarded children do not respond. The degree of neuropathic insult, then, measured in terms of intellectual capacity, predicts the success of treatment with a presynaptic agonist. Yet, among moderately and severely retarded subjects, we find amantadine responders. When axial, brain-stem structures are impaired, whatever hope one may have of success can come only by way of directly stimulating the postsynaptic neuron.

REFERENCES

Alexandris A, Lundell FN: Effect of thioridazine, amphetamine and placebo on the hyperkinetic syndrome and cognitive area in mental deficient children. Can Med Assoc J 98:92–96, 1968

Allen RM: Palliative treatment of tardive dyskinesia with combination of amantadine-neuroleptic administration. Biol Psychiatry 17:719–727, 1982

Allen RM: Role of amantadine in the management of neuroleptic-induced extrapyramidal syndromes: overview and pharmacology. Clinical Neuropharmacology 6:564–573, 1983

Aman MG: Stimulant drug effects in developmental disorders and hyperactivity—toward a resolution of disparate findings. J Autism Dev Disord 12:385–398, 1982

Aman MG, Singh NN: Methylphenidate in severely retarded residents and the clinical significance of stereotypic behavior. Appl Res Ment Retard 3:345–358, 1982

Ambrosini PJ, Fried J: Preliminary report: amantadine hydrochloride in childhood enuresis. J Clin Psychopharmacol 4:223–235, 1984

Ananth J, Sangani H, Noonan JPA: Amantadine therapy for drug induced extrapyramidal signs and depression. Psychiatry J Univ Ottawa 1:27–33, 1977

Angrist B, Rotrosen J, Gershon S: Differential effects of amphetamine and neuroleptics on negative vs. positive symptoms in schizophrenia. Psychopharmacology 72:17–18, 1980

Aoki FY, Sitar DS: Clinical pharmacokinetics of amantadine hydrochloride. Clin Pharmacokinet 14:35–51, 1988

Aoki FY, Sitar DS: Amantadine kinetics in healthy elderly men: implications for influenza prevention. Clin Pharmacol Ther 37:137–144, 1985

Aoki FY, Stiver HG, Sitar DS, et al: Prophylactic amantadine dose and plasma concentration-effect relationships in healthy adults. Clin Pharmacol Ther 37:128–136, 1985

Bailey EV, Stone TW: The mechanism of action of amantadine in Parkinsonism: a review. Arch Internat Pharmacodyn 216:248, 1975

Bean B: Antiviral therapy: new drugs and their uses. Postgrad Medicine 80:109–120, 1986

Beleslin DB, Samardzic R, Stefanovic-Denic K: 6-Hydroxydopamine and aggression in cats. Pharmacology Biochemistry and Behavior 14 (suppl 1):29–32, 1981

Bell A, Zubek JP: Effects of Deanol on the intellectual performance of mental defectives. Can J Psychol 15:172–175, 1961

Blacklidge VY, Ekblad RL: The effectiveness of methylphenidate hydrochloride (Ritalin) on learning and behavior in public school educable mentally retarded children. Pediatrics 47:923–926, 1971

Bleidner WE, Harmon JB, Hewes WE, et al: Absorption, distribution and excretion of amantadine. J Pharmacol Exp Ther 150:484–490, 1965

Borison RL: Amantadine-induced psychosis in a geriatric patient with renal disease. Am J Psychiatry 136:111–112, 1979

Borison RL: Amantadine in the management of extrapyramidal side effects. Clinical Neuropharmacology 6:557–563, 1983

Borison RL, Davis JM: Amantadine in Tourette syndrome. Current Psychiatric Therapies 22:127–130, 1983

Braham J: Jacob-Creutzfeldt disease: treatment by amantadine. Br Med J 4:212–213, 1971

Campbell M: Pharmacotherapy in early infantile autism. Biol Psychiatry 10:399–423, 1975

Chandler MC, Barnhill JL, Gualtieri CT: Amantadine for the agitated head-injury patient. Brain Injury 2(4):309–311, 1988

Cox B, Tha SJ: Effects of amantadine and l-dopa on apomorphine- and *d*-amphetamine-induced stereotyped behavior in rats. Eur J Pharmacol 24:96–100, 1973

Dales S, Choppin PW: Attachment and penetration of influenza virus. Virology 18:489–492, 1962

Davidoff E, Reifenstein EC: Treatment of schizophrenia with sympatho-mimetic drugs: benzedrine sulfate. Psychiatr Q 13:127–144, 1939

Davies WL, Grunert RR, Haff RF, et al: Antiviral activity of *l*-adaman-tanamine (amantadine). Science 144:862–863, 1964

Davis KV, Sprague RL, Werry JS: Stereotyped behavior and activity level in severe retardates: the effects of drugs. Am J Ment Defic 73:721–727, 1969

Evans RW, Gualtieri CT: Stimulant effects in closed head injury patients. Paper presented at the annual meeting of the International Neuro-psychological Society, Washington, DC, 1987

Fann WE, Lake CR: Amantadine vs. trihexyphenidyl in the treatment of drug-induced Parkinsonism. Am J Psychiatry 133:940–943, 1976

Feeney DM, Gonzalez A, Law WA: Amphetamine, haloperidol and ex-perience interact to affect rate of recovery after motor cortex injury. Science 217:855–857, 1982

Fleet WS, Valenstein E, Watson RT, et al: Dopamine agonist therapy for neglect in humans. Neurology 37:1765–1770, 1987

Fleischhacker WW, Buchgeher A, Schubert H: Mematine in the treatment of senile dementia of the Alzheimer type. Prog Neuropsychopharmacol Biol Psychiatry 10:89–93, 1986

Galbraith AW, Oxford JS, Schild GC, et al: Study of l-adamantanamine hydrochloride used prophylactically during the Hong Kong influenza epidemic in a family environment. Bull WORLD Health Organ 41:677–682, 1969

Gelenberg AJ: Amantadine in the treatment of benzotropine-refractory extrapyramidal disorders induced by antipsychotic drugs. Curr Ther Res 23:375–380, 1978

Gelenberg AJ, Mandel MR: Catatonic reactions to high-potency neuroleptic drugs. Arch Gen Psychiatry 34:947–950, 1977

Gianutsos G, Stewart C, Dunn JP: Pharmacological changes in dopaminergic systems induced by long-term administration of amantadine. Eur J Pharmacol 110:357–361, 1985

Granato JE, Stern BJ, Ringel A, et al: Neuroleptic malignant syndrome: successful treatment with dantrolene and bromocriptine. Ann Neurol 14:89–90, 1983

Gualtieri CT: Pharmacotherapy and the neurobehavioral sequelae of traumatic brain injury. Brain Injury (in press)

Gualtieri CT, Evans RW: Stimulant treatment for the neurobehavioral sequelae of traumatic brain injury. Brain Injury 2:273–290, 1988

Hamburg P, Weilburg JB, Cassem NH, et al: Relapse of neuroleptic malignant syndrome with early discontinuation of amantadine therapy. Compr Psychiatry 27:272–275, 1986

Harper RW, Knothe UC: Coloured Lilliputian hallucinations with amantadine. Med J Aust 1:444–445, 1973

Harvey NS: Psychiatric disorders in Parkinsonism, 2: organic cerebral states and drug reactions. Psychosomatics 27:177–184, 1986

Hordam VW, Sharp JG, Smilack JD, et al: Pharmacokinetics of amantadine hydrochloride in subjects with normal impaired renal function. Ann Intern Med 94:454–458, 1981

Ing TS, Daugirdas JT, Soung LS, et al: Toxic effects of amantadine in patients with renal failure. Can Med Assoc J 120:695–698, 1979

Janowsky DS, Serkeke HJ, Davis JM: Differential effects of amantadine on pseudoparkinsonism and tardive dyskinesia. Psychopharmacol Bull 9:11–15, 1973

Kelley JT, Abuzzahab FS: The antiparkinson properties of amantadine in drug-induced Parkinsonism. J Clin Pharmacol 11:211–214, 1971

Koppel C, Tenczer J: A revision of the metabolic disposition of amantadine. Biochemical Mass Spectrometry 12:497–501, 1985

Kornetsky C: Hyporesponsivity of chronic schizophrenic patients to dextroamphetamine. Arch Gen Psychiatry 33:1425–1428, 1976

Lazarus A: Treating neuroleptic malignant syndrome. Am J Psychiatry 141:1014–1015, 1984

Livingston S, Kajdi L, Bridge E: The use of benzedrine and dexedrine sulfate in the treatment of epilepsy. J Pediatrics 32:490–494, 1948

Lungberg T, Ungerstedt U: Reinstatement of eating by dopamine agonist in aphagic dopamine denervated rats. Physiol Behav 17:817–822, 1976

Maeda H, Maki S: Dopamine agonists produce functional recovery from septal lesions which affect hypothalmic defensive attack in cats. Brain Res 407(2):381–385, 1987

Marotta RF, Potegal M, Glusman M, et al: Dopamine agonists induce recovery from surgically-induced septal rage. Nature 269:513–515, 1977

Marshall JF, Gotthelf T: Sensory inattention in rats with 6-hydroxy-dopamine-induced degeneration of ascending dopaminergic neurons: apomorphine-induced reversal of deficits. Exp Neurol 65:398–411, 1979

Marshall JF, Ungerstedt U: Apomophine-induced restoration of drinking to thirst challenges in 6-hydroxydopamine-treated rats. Physiol Behav 17:817–822, 1976

Mattes J: A pilot trial of amantadine in hyperactive children. Psychology Bulletin 16:67–69, 1980

McEvoy JP, McCue M, Spring B, et al: Effects of amantadine and trihexyphenidyl on memory in elderly normal volunteers. Am J Psychiatry 144:573–577, 1987

Meldrum BS, Turski L, Schwarz M, et al: Anticonvulsant action of 1,3-dimethyl-5-aminoadamantane: pharmacological studies in rodents and baboon. Papio Papio, Naunyn Schmiedebergs Arch Pharmacol 332: 93–97, 1986

Menon MK, Clark WG, Fleming RM: Blockade of the central effects of *d*-amphetamine sulfate by amantadine hydrochloride. Eur J Pharmacol 21:311–317, 1973

Menon MK, Vivonia CA, Haddox VG: Evidence for presynaptic antagonism by amantadine of indirectly acting central stimulants. Psychopharmacology 83:89–91, 1984

Messiha FS: Antagonism of ethanol-evoked responses by amantadine: a possible clinical application: pharmacology. Biochemistry and Behavior 8:573–577, 1978

Millet VM, Diesbach M, Bryson YJ: Double-blind controlled study of central nervous system side effects of amantadine hydrochloride, rimantadine hydrochloride and chlorpheniramine. Antimicrob Agents Chemother 21:1–4, 1982

Mlele TJ, Wiley YV: Clopenthixol decanoate in the management of aggressive mentally handicapped patients. Br J Psychiatry 149:373–376, 1986

MMWR: Antiviral agents for influenza A. JAMA 258:599–600, 1987

Muller HF, Dastoor DP, Klinger A, et al: Amantadine in senile dementia: electroencephalographic and clinical effects. J Geriatrics Society 27:9–16, 1979

Murray TJ: Amantadine therapy for fatigue in multiple sclerosis. Can J Neurol Sci 12:251–254, 1985

Nestlebaum Z, Siris SG, Rifkin A, et al: Exacerbation of schizophrenia with amantadine. Am J Psychiatry 143:1170–1171, 1986

Papeschi R: Amantadine may stimulate dopamine and noradrenalin receptors. Neuropharmacology 13:77–83, 1974

Postma JU, Van Tilburg W: Visual hallucinations and delirium during treatment with amantadine (Symmetrel). J Am Geriatr Soc 23:212–215, 1975

Pradhan SN: Aggression and central neurotransmitters. Int Rev Neurobiol 18:213–262, 1975

Prepas S, Menon MK, Clark WG: Blockade of the central effects of *d*-amphetamine by amantadine, II: drug research. Arzneimittel forschung 25:780–782, 1985

Reines ED, Gross PA: Antiviral agents. Med Clin North Am 72:691–715, 1988

Reiser G, Binmoller FJ, Koch R: Memantine (1-amino-3-5-dimethyladamantane) blocks the serotonin induced depolarization response in a neuronal cell line. Brain Research 443:338–344, 1988

Rizzo M, Morselli PL: Amantadine-induced aggressiveness. Br Med J 3:50, 1972

Ross ED, Stewart RM: Akinetic mutism from hypothalamic damage: successful treatment with dopamine agonists. Neurology 31:1435–1439, 1981

Safta L, Cuparencu B, Danau M, et al: Some behavioral changes induced by amantadine (adamantine). Acta Biol Med Germ 35(2):229–233, 1976

Sartori M, Pratt CM, Young JB: Torsade de Pointe: malignant cardiac arrhythmia induced by amantadine poisoning. Am J Med 77:388–391, 1984

Schneiden H, Cox B: A comparison between amantadine and bromocriptine using the Stereotyped Behavior Response test (SBR) in the rat. Eur J Pharmacol 39:133–141, 1976

Schwab RS, England AC, Poskanzer DC, et al: Amantadine in the treatment of Parkinson's disease. JAMA 208:1168–1170, 1969

Schwab RS, Poskanzer DC, England AC, et al: Amantadine in Parkinson's disease: review of more than two years experience. JAMA 222:792–795, 1972

Shealy CN, Weeth JB, Mercier D: Livedo reticularis in patients with parkinsonism receiving amantadine. JAMA 212:1522–1523, 1970

Shields WD, Lake JL, Chugani HT: Amantadine in the treatment of refractory epilepsy in childhood: an open trial in 10 patients. Neurology 35:579–581, 1985

Siever LJ: The effect of amantadine on prolactin levels and galactorrhea on neuroleptic-treated patients. J Clin Psychopharmacol 1:2–7, 1981

Simpson DM, David GC: Dopamine agonist and neuroleptic malignant syndrome. Am J Psychiatry 142:270–271, 1985

Stenson RL, Donlon PT, Meyer JE: Comparison of benzotropine mesylate and amantadine HCl in neuroleptic-induced extrapyramidal symptoms. Compr Psychiatry 17:763–768, 1976

Stetter H: The chemistry of the organic ring systems with urotropine structure. Angew Chem 66:217–229, 1954

Stromberg U, Svensson TH, Waldeck B: On the mode of action amantadine. J Pharm Pharmacol 22:959–962, 1970

Van Putten T, Gelenberg AJ, Lavori PW, et al: Anticholinergic effects on memory: benztropine vs. amantadine. Psychopharmacol Bull 23:26–29, 1987

Vardi J, Streifler M: On the synchronizing effect of amantadine-1-

hydrochloric (Symmetrel) on pathological EEG-activity. J Neural Transmission 37:73, 1975

Varley CK, Trupin EW: Double blind administration of methylphenidate to mentally retarded children with attention deficit disorder: a preliminary study. Am J Ment Defic 86:560–566, 1982

Vollum DI, Parkes JD, Doyle D: Livedo reticularis during amantadine treatment. Br Med J 2:627–682, 1971

Wilson TW, Rajput AH: Amantadine-dyazide interaction. Can Med Assoc J 129:974–975, 1983

Wu MJ, Ing TS, Soung LS, et al: Amantadine hydrochloride pharmacokinetics in patients with impaired renal function. Clinical Nephrology 17:19–23, 1982

Zubenko G, Pope HG, Jr: Management of a case of neuroleptic malignant syndrome with bromocriptine. Am J Psychiatry 140:1619–1620, 1983